BEFORE
THE
TIME
COMES

Have a Senior Conversation,

Monica

MONICA E. YOUNG

BEFORE THE TIME COMES
Conversations Family Caregivers Need to Have With Their Elderly Parents—A Senior Living Guide

MONICA E. YOUNG

PUBLISHED BY
www.MonicaEYoung.com

ISBN 978-1-7350810-0-7

Contact the author at meyoungauthor@gmail.com

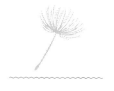

PRAISE

Monica, You are great! I talked to Ardis tonight, and she seemed so pleased with the move. We are in NM heading for AZ tomorrow. This has been so easy from afar with your help. Thanks again.

—BARRY SWANSON

Monica, When I saw the emailed photos of my aunt's new place, I thought I was looking at her old house—excellent job! Wow ... how beautiful. I can't believe so much fit into that apt. You're a miracle worker ☺ Thanks so much.

—KRIS CUOMO

Dear Monica, Thank you so very much for the wonderful moving experience. You all are wonderful! Many, many thanks. Cheers!

**—DODI, SUSIE, CHARLIE, AND CARL ("THE KIDS")
FOR ANITA FREDERICKS ("THE MOM")**

Monica, Thank you for helping me with Ralph's move. I appreciate your efficiency and how easy you made the move for me.

—DARLENE CLARK

Dear Monica, I ended up [moving mom from independent living to assisted living] myself. It took me three days! I don't care what you charge. It's worth it.

—BILL (LAST NAME UNKNOWN)

Dear Monica, A note of thanks doesn't seem like enough …. You made a difficult time so easy. Things could not have gone better. Your ladies are great gals! We will highly recommend your services to others.

—SINCERELY, EILEEN CANOVATCHEL

Dear Monica, Thank you for your thoughtful and caring touch in moving my dad last year and again in May. You have made this last transition much easier for all of us. I know my dad truly appreciated all of your care.

—STEVE PROUT

Monica, The move was awesome … but the way you treated my parents—that's what makes you a professional!

—PATRICIA

Dear Monica & Staff, On behalf of our family, we would like to thank you for several days of work. We could not make the connections without your help. You were right; it was an emotional time. We are all back home now and dealing with the loss. Just wanted to thank you for stepping up to the task.

—JOHN REINITZ & FAMILY

Dear Monica, You did such a "great" job moving me. I wish you a very happy and successful fifth year.

—DOROTHY MCGOWAN

Monica, I will never forget all you did to help Mom and me and my family. You are an angel! And so are all of your team members! You treated us with such dignity during a very tough time. I miss my mom so much, you can't imagine. But it was such a blessing to have your help in dealing with all the things. God bless you. Thanks for all your work & caring!

—SUSAN CROFTON

Monica, Everyone is **raving** *about how well your team worked packing and unpacking, and how great the apt. looks. I appreciate the photos and I can now* **rave** *also! Mom seems very happy with her things and is busy getting acclimated. The staff at the community all came in to look at the magic you created. They emailed me as to how wonderful everything looks, and they all loved the paint-*

ings you hung! Then my mom's neighbors came over and repeated the above sentiments! Even my brother Rob and his wife, Janinne, said that they couldn't believe how quick/efficient/and great you all were! They were astonished on your attention to detail! So rave reviews all the way around! You are great at what you do! I am so glad the community referred you! You can use this email as a testimony on your website!

—SUZANNE, FOR FAMILY OF MARY FRANCES JACOBS

CONTENTS

DEDICATED TO OUR FAMILY TEAM:

Ellen, Agnes, Mary, Cathy,
Monica, Marian ... and Mother

THE RING

A wedding ring,

A symbol of love,

At death, a treasure for the living.

Who can claim it?

Who should claim it?

A journey among the six sisters begins.

An excuse to renew the family bonds.

From oldest to youngest,

Its journey continues.

It travels on over the years.

Forged by an uncle,

Worn by a mother,

Her hands always bearing its weight,

Twisting as the fingers age,

Resting on her heart at the end.

For twenty years, it has continued to live.

On the hands of the sisters,

In the hearts of the sisters.

A symbol of togetherness,

A symbol of love.

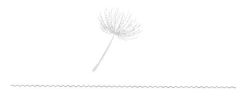

INTRODUCTION

Help! After helping more than a thousand families negotiate transitions with their aging parents, *help* was the word I heard over and over again when families first engaged my services. Most often, they would come as the result of a crisis triggered by health or time commitments or both.

So why is it that while aging is a fact of life, it comes as a surprise that our parents need to be cared for? Why do we avoid the subject only to find ourselves in crisis mode? What are we supposed to do? And how are we supposed to do it?

Such questions led me to start my senior move management business in 2005. The answers to these questions gained through well over a decade of helping seniors and families make informed and compassionate decisions for the next stage of life led to writing this book. The goal is to make the critical information and important resources found within available to even more families in the most timely manner possible. There is much to share with you, but first I would like to briefly tell you my family history and the stories of my first and last clients as they so clearly demonstrate both the strong need for planning as well as what motivated me to get started in this business helping families.

My mother lived alone in Baltimore. The rest of our family was scattered across the United States. After my mom suffered several falls (and I made several trips back east), we realized it was time to do something. The diagnosis of Alzheimer's moved our decision-making and helping into high gear. An assisted living community that met our standards had an opening. How could we afford it? Selling the house was the obvious answer. Thus began my first job as a senior move manager. My five sisters and I would work together to complete the monumental task of emptying the house my dad had built in 1938. We each had one week of vacation. Was that enough time? As it turns out, it wasn't.

But the seeds of helping others in the same situation had been planted, and so much knowledge had been gained by struggling through this experience. Surely I could make it easier for other children of aging parents! Enter Minnie and Robert, my first clients (names have been changed).

Minnie was a military officer's wife, an important distinction in her and her family's world because it encompassed an array of duties required to support her officer husband. Her move needed to mirror what she had experienced in her frequent military moves, and her children were working full time and were pretty much unavailable to help. In true military style, Minnie took charge and introduced me to the importance of space planning. Blue masking tape became an essential in my toolkit, my box of basics, thanks to her insistence that we diagram each piece of furniture in its new location in the new apartment. She also taught me patience because, after three attempts, the bed was still not made correctly.

Minnie and Robert had recognized that their physical limitations were making yardwork and housework too hard. An independent living community offered relief from those responsibilities. My company offered a new and better way to move because it included complete packing and unpacking services. When we left their new "home," everything had been put away, clocks were set to the correct time, and pictures were hung; in essence, their new situation mirrored their previous one as much as possible, and they could feel at home and in control right away. This move took five days to complete, and my business partner and I learned a lot.

My final move was for Cathy. Over the years, my company had been called upon by her family six different times, as circumstances changed. When I first met them, Cathy and her mother were living together because they each had limitations best addressed by this mutual care-giving relationship. When Cathy married, she and her mother both wanted to remain within close proximity to each other which made a move to a cottage in the same community a great solution.

Once again, my company assisted in moving, packing, and unpacking, a process refined to the point that a move could be completed in one day. Then Cathy's husband died, so Cathy and her mother moved back in together. After her mother's death, Cathy insisted that I help her move to truly independent living, a house of her own.

Of the many things I learned from Cathy and her mother, perhaps the one that stands out the most is of what true family means. Their demonstration of a caring and loving relationship that survived through years of emotional changes is a lesson I cherish. By watching and sharing in their planning and the ways they cared for each other, I developed key ideas that every family needs to consider to help make these life transitions go smoothly and as stress-free as possible.

In case you can't tell, I loved and learned from my senior move management business and from those families who entrusted themselves to my company's care. The insights gained over those eleven years form the values presented in this book. I share them with you in the hopes that you will embrace your family's end-of-life journey.

My mission statement said the goal was "To transition seniors, and/or their families, comfortably, efficiently, and lovingly into the next stage of their lives." If you'd like to take your own family through this transition, this book of ideas can help "Before the Time Comes."

LEARN THE TERMINOLOGY

As with most industries, senior care workers have developed a language to simplify communication. In the following pages, some of this shorthand will be explained in depth. Don't be shy about asking questions when confronted by these new and strange expressions.

One of the oddest comments for me was when I overheard a nurse saying to another nurse, "They'll probably need to go to a skaniff."

My brain understood that they were referring to the dreaded nursing home. Only after hearing this same comment several times did I ask and learn the correct term—SNF.

No longer is *nursing home* an acceptable reference. (Thank goodness for that!) A SNF is a *skilled nursing facility*, sometimes pronounced *ska-niff*. The reason for the change is to assure patients that the intention is for them to leave. Needing skilled care is, most likely, a temporary situation. As long as patients continue to improve, they can plan to return to their previous situation. The long-term solution means going home, not staying in a home.

Becoming familiar with the following acronyms can help you navigate the process:

- CCRC—CONTINUING CARE RETIREMENT COMMUNITY

- IL—INDEPENDENT LIVING

- AL—ASSISTED LIVING

- SNF—SKILLED NURSING FACILITY

- IHSS—IN-HOME SUPPORTIVE SERVICES

- ADL—ACTIVITIES OF DAILY LIVING

- IADL—INSTRUMENTAL ACTIVITIES OF DAILY LIVING

- UTI—URINARY TRACT INFECTION

- DNR—DO NOT RESUSCITATE

- MD POA—MEDICAL POWER OF ATTORNEY

- POA—POWER OF ATTORNEY (FOR FINANCIAL REASONS)

- POD—PAYABLE ON DEATH

- HIPAA—HEALTH INSURANCE PORTABILITY AND ACCOUNTABILITY ACT OF 1996 (FEDERAL LAW PROTECTING PRIVACY OF PATIENT RECORDS)

My contribution:

- F.A.S.T.—FAMILY, ARGH, SELL, TRASH (MY METHOD OF SORTING)

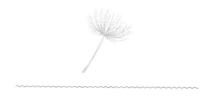

HOW TO USE
THIS GUIDE

This guide was created to be a nontechnical and very practical resource for everyone. When I talk about you, I mean you, the reader; you, the senior; and/or you, the family team member. For your consideration and enlightenment, I've tried to identify all the roles needed.

There are five steps or five decision-partner roles. These roles include:

- MAKING A PLAN

- CHOOSING A NEW HOME

- TAKING CARE OF THE PERSON

- COLLECTING ESSENTIAL PAPERWORK

- RECORDING THE LEGACY

The lead statement on my original website was "Dying is a fact of life, so why are we so often surprised by it?" The answer seems to be because we don't want to face it. After assisting so many seniors who *have* faced it, my conscience tells me that now is the time to share what I have learned. Can you and your family share the end-of-life-journey in a graceful manner? Use this guide; many of these suggestions will help.

The chapter list in the Contents serves as a way to go directly to the subject that concerns you most. Alternatively, you should consider reading this book in the order in which it is presented. The five steps are in a sequence that makes sense based on my experience as a senior move manager. However, the steps can be completed in any order.

The workbook format is supported by examples and summaries at the end of each subchapter. These exercises will reinforce concrete concepts and stimulate your own thoughts with the goal of creating your own path forward.

Some of you will consider reading this book because you're in an emergency situation. The "Need to Do It Now" plan (sub section at beginning of Chapter 3) provides the "quick and dirty" steps to get you through this *Oh, NO* attempt to take control.

Chapter 2, "Having the Senior Conversation" and Chapter 3, "Making a Plan," especially "The Long-Term Plan," are the ultimate control solutions. If you do nothing else, read these two chapters.

"Choosing a New Home" in Chapter 4 provides easy-to-use suggestions for those making "The Middle Ground Plan" as well as those making "The Long-Term Plan," both found in Chapter 3.

"Taking Care of the Person" in Chapter 5 translates to managing expectations on what is humanly possible, compared to what is best for all. Burnout is very real.

By "Collecting Essential Paperwork" (Chapter 6), your team will acquire the peace of mind that comes from knowing where things stand as of this moment.

By "Recording the Legacy" (Chapter 7), a look at the past, your comfort level will increase even more.

Of course this comfort will be tested when there is a sudden change in plans. I'm not trying to scare you. I'm just trying to let you know that even the best of plans might not work. Anticipate changes.

Confronting the end is always painful. Even though my mother passed away in 2002, there are still times when a memory of her will bring tears to my eyes. Writing this guide has brought so many of these memories. You'll probably experience a wide range of emotions as you prepare yourselves. And you'll never be completely prepared, no matter how much you plan.

A final note. Depending on the topic, I direct my concerns to the decision maker. During my career as a senior move manager, about half the time the senior was the one pushing for decisions; the other half of the time the family team was doing the pushing. Ultimately, the whole team accepted the natural progression to the next stage. Use this guide to lead you on that same journey.

REMOVING THE BLINDERS

When you see a person on a daily basis, you tend to miss the subtle changes occurring. Time-lapse photography is a good example of what I'm trying to make you *see*. What does each person look like today, and only today?

Think about hanging a picture. You position it, you hang it, then you adjust it. A little later, you may adjust it again. Over time, you continue to glance at it occasionally. It becomes a constant in your daily routine. But do you see it in the same way you did originally? Do you notice the dust on the top and around the edges? Life, and your loved one, are kind of like that picture, over time. Look at the person in front of you with fresh eyes. I'm not trying to tell you to judge this person so much as suggesting you evaluate what you see.

Try this exercise first: Stand in front of a mirror. Close your eyes. Empty your mind's eye. In other words, forget how you want to look. Forget how you think you look. Pretend you are going to see yourself, "warts and all"? When you're ready, open your eyes. Now you can see the real you. I call this exercise "Removing the Blinders" because I want you to free your mind from past perceptions. Past perceptions can blind you to what is being presented today. Look anew. Be ready to say, "So this is me."

In the same way, you can remove the blinders and truly see your family member. Time has inevitably changed this person, just as it has changed you. Are you ready? It's time to pay an important visit to your loved one, with your eyes open. Follow these steps:

1.   STAND OUTSIDE THE FRONT DOOR.

2.   TAKE A DEEP BREATH.

3.   REMOVE ANY EXPECTATIONS.

4.   STEP INSIDE WITH YOUR EYES WIDE OPEN.

5.   TAKE MENTAL PICTURES.

6.   EVALUATE AFTER LEAVING.

The results of this evaluation can and should take some time. I like to let my subconscious mind guide me when making hard decisions. Are you ready to become an informed and helpful decision partner for your senior family member?

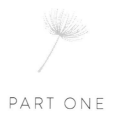

PART ONE

PLANNING FOR A SENIOR MOVE

'm reminded of the adage, "No time like the present." You might be considering the direction in which life is heading. This thought has probably been triggered by a recent event. Or maybe an accumulation of triggers combined to let you know that the time to reevaluate circumstances should be now. Perhaps the results of the removing the blinders exercise have hit home. Let's talk about what those triggers are saying.

External triggers are gentle reminders that life has an end. The death of a friend or loved one always prompts a look at your own life. Birthdays are just a number, but as a friend recently said, "If I'm fifty-two, that means my mom is seventy-two!" Are you ready for life's end? Another, less personal gotcha: Medicare at sixty-five; Social Security at sixty-six (or soon thereafter). Ageism is a fact of life, as represented by these numbers. No offense intended. External triggers allow time to make decisions.

Internal triggers are more insistent. A callback after a recent doctor's exam for more testing. Catching the flu or suffering an injury, both of which take weeks or months to recover from. Internal triggers say, *Do it now*. That inner voice wants to be heard.

Whatever factors have caused this evaluation, know that you and your team are ultimately in control. I know that asking for help doesn't come easily to those who feel independent and self-assured. In the course of my Senior Move Manager® (SMM) business life, I met many of you, along with your equally independent, self-assured, and quite-capable-of-handling-things family members. I want to share two different journeys by two independent seniors whom I had the pleasure of knowing during the course of my career. They and their families chose different solutions. Adjusting expectations to fit evolving situations will be an ongoing effort. Consider which goal your family team might choose.

It still makes me smile to think of the woman who said she was going to stay home and die with all her beautiful things. She had accumulated art and furniture to be marveled at. The view from her home was a beautiful overlook. After spending some time enjoying her home, and getting to know her, I realized she had made a decision that suited her personality.

Another strong woman contacted me with a different approach. Her decision led her to move into a senior community for the last year of her life. Again, an independent, strong-willed senior. She had also accumulated art and furniture to be marveled at. But her family lived out of state, so she typically handled things on her own. She too had made a decision that suited her personality.

Where are you and your family team on this journey? How much independence is possible? What decision will suit your personality? How involved will your family be? Can you let them help? By reading "Making the Team" and "Having the Senior Conversation," these questions will begin to be answered.

The following checklist will help you and your family start this journey together. (Note: While I like to have at least three choices at all times, this number can vary.)

REFERENCES YOU'LL WANT

- CHOICES FOR REHAB (3)

- CHOICES FOR SENIOR LIVING COMMUNITIES (3)

- CHOICES FOR HOME CARE (3)

- CLEANING PERSON: REGULAR

- CLEANING PERSON: DEEP CLEANING

- ESTATE ATTORNEY

- CERTIFIED PUBLIC ACCOUNTANT (CPA)

- HEALTH COMPANION

- FINANCIAL ADVISOR

- SENIOR MOVE MANAGER

- APPRAISER

- AUCTION HOUSE

- ESTATE SALES COMPANY

- DONATION PICKUP

- JUNK REMOVAL/SHREDDING SERVICE

- REALTOR

- GUN SELLER

- JEWELRY BUYER

- COINS/PRECIOUS METALS BUYER

- FUNERAL DIRECTOR

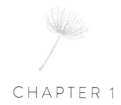

CHAPTER 1

MAKING THE TEAM

Our journey started with a broken hip. It often does. Time to help our mother ease into the final stage of life; that is, growing old gracefully—with help.

The team had come into existence, imperceptibly, over time. In our family's case, it had happened over a period spanning some twenty years. Looking back, one could say it began with the long, painful death of our father (from cancer), at the age of sixty-nine.

Step One became arranging a funeral. Because our parents had spent their whole lives in the same area of a large city, choosing a funeral director was almost easy. Many of their friends' arrangements had been handled by this same service. Picking a casket was not so easy. The price ranges were surprising. Suffice it to say that "shopping" for a casket after the death of a loved one is *not* the best time to make that decision. A prearranged funeral service became Step One for our team.

At some point, several years later, one of us noticed unpaid bills at our mother's house. My husband and I introduced the idea of getting my mother's legal and financial affairs in proper order. My mother welcomed this concept and set about making it happen. My husband located an estate attorney in the state where my mother lived, as state laws vary. This attorney handled the will and setting up a trust. That was Step Two.

Next was the fall. *Why isn't she answering the phone? I know she's there.* Mother was lying on the floor by the front door. She wasn't responding to the doorbell, or the knocking, or the repeated "Mother, are you OK?" After trying the back door and considering breaking a window, the decision to break the chain on the front door allowed entry. Mother had fallen asleep, uninjured, where she lay. Repeated attempts to get up had proven useless, so she had eventually given in to the need to rest. We decided she couldn't live alone—Step Three.

Our family of seven children had one member who readily volunteered—volunteered to give up her current life, move back to the family home, and become the daily caregiver for our mother. Another family member took on the task of remodeling this same home to add a half bath on the main level. The dining room became the bedroom. Step Four, also known as supporting the desire to remain at home as long as possible, accomplished.

* * *

All she did was go out to get the mail. Can you imagine the horror you feel when you are told by your mother's neighbor that your mother is lying in the front yard? The doctor tries to console you by saying that, at eighty-five years of age, a hip often fractures, followed by the fall.

Decisions about surgery and rehab followed. Two members with medical POA conferred. Rehab was in the rehab care center next to the hospital. Step Five was complete, but the team was only partially ready.

And so began the last five years of our mother's life. Complications were many. The largest was finding a safe place for her to stay (at least three care locations were tried and deemed unacceptable). Her second broken hip, combined with the beginnings of dementia, were painful times for all of us. The need to sell the house—the family home—took time and devotion. Another member arranged the sale—Step Six. The team did OK, considering. Why weren't we better prepared?

This guide is being written because after this experience with my parents, then a similar experience with my in-laws, I began a senior move manager business. Based on personal experience and more than one thousand experiences with other seniors, I hope to give you the tools to prepare for the end of life's journey. It's going to happen. It's time to face it with resolve and acceptance. Your choice, and your team's choice, can be to handle it with grace. My choice is to help you make this happen. It's time to make the team and start planning how to help.

Steps for the Family

1. MAKE THE TEAM.

2. HAVE THE CONVERSATION.

3. ASSIGN TASKS.

4. COMMUNICATE STATUS.

5. BE READY.

6. ANTICIPATE CHANGES.

Steps for the Senior

1. PREARRANGE FUNERAL.

2. COMPLETE LEGAL PIECES.

3. ANALYZE LIVING ALONE.

4. CHOOSE A REHAB CENTER (BEFORE IT'S NEEDED).

5. CHOOSE A COMMUNITY.

6. SELL AND EMPTY THE HOME.

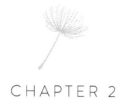

CHAPTER 2

HAVING THE SENIOR
CONVERSATION

People ask me all the time, "What's the right age to move into a retirement community?" The average age of the seniors I moved was eighty-five. Is that the right age? It depends.

Remember our previous discussion about internal and external triggers? Let's continue with the evaluation you came to after "Removing the Blinders." Your grandparents, your parents, or your loved ones seem to be OK with their living situation. What you notice is what you consider to be too much dust. Old newspapers are accumulating by the recliner, which presents a safety hazard. "Final Notice" catches your eye as you go by the pile of mail on the desk in the kitchen. What should you do?

It's time to have the "Senior Conversation." How that looks depends on who initiates the discussion. Emotions will be fragile. Keep this in mind.

THE SENIOR'S PERSPECTIVE

As gently and kindly as possible, ask all of your likely team members when it would be a good time to have a serious discussion with them. (No minor children.) Their answer will determine where you go from here. A positive answer might be, "We can talk about it, if you really want to." Now is the time for firm emphasis that this meeting must happen. A negative answer, such as "Oh, Mom (or Dad), you're not going to die any time soon," means that they're trying to protect themselves from facing the future. Given enough time, as well as repeated requests, the answer becomes, "Wow, you're serious. What would you like me to do?" Be ready to put your thoughts and emotions into words. "I want to move ahead, but I can't do it without your help."

THE TEAM'S PERSPECTIVE

As gently and kindly as possible, ask if you can talk about what the next five years looks like to your loved one. Their answer will determine where you go from here. A positive answer might be "Well, honey, I just haven't thought about it." This answer provides an opening for you. A negative answer, such as "Don't worry about me. I'll let you know when I need your help," is an attempt to stop the discussion before it starts. The answer you will probably hear is, "We plan to stay in the house as long as possible. And when the time comes, we'll move to one of those retirement places like so-and-so did. Why do you ask?"

Let's examine why you should ask, and what you expect to accomplish.

Consensus and team building are your goals. Basically, you want to have a plan, and you want it to be a team plan. Emphasize that it needs to be a team plan. You can and will help, when the time comes. You just don't want the time to come and not know what the plan is. Kind, gentle concern is all you are going to communicate at this juncture. You want to be part of the team, and you want to know the plan.

Who should be the person to initiate this discussion? If you've had your family's "Making the Team" discussion, perhaps you've already chosen the lead team member for this step on the journey. Although I'm calling it "Having the Senior Conversation," in reality, it will take many conversations to come up with a best solution. And other team members will probably want to have their own conversations before a group decision is made. This is consensus building in the best way possible.

So what happens if you *don't* have the conversation now? The "Need to Do It Now" plan focuses on this unfortunate position. Having the senior conversation may be hard, but *not* having a plan is so much harder. Better to take control now. And now will require several conversations. And the plan will come together several conversations later.

One more caveat. Should the question of moving to a retirement community come up, your comment should be, "That may be one option." In so many ways, I don't believe the time to broach this subject is while having the senior conversation. Steer the thoughts and ideas back to "What do you think you want to do?" and "How can we help?"

CONVERSATION DOS AND DON'TS

- DO LISTEN INTENTLY.

- DO ASK QUESTIONS.

- DO EXPRESS YOUR CONCERNS.

- DO SAY THAT YOU WANT TO HELP.

- DO SAY THAT YOU NEED TO HELP.

- DON'T OFFER ADVICE.

- DON'T ALLOW THE CONVERSATION TO GO ASTRAY.

- DON'T DISCUSS MOVING (EVEN IF THE IDEA IS MENTIONED).

- DON'T HAVE THIS DISCUSSION WHILE YOUR LOVED ONE IS ILL OR HURTING.

- DON'T EVER USE THE WORD "FACILITY" IN ANY CONVERSATION.

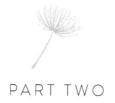

PART TWO

THE FIVE
ESSENTIALS

You're probably asking yourself, "Yeah, but where do I start?" Believe me, I really wanted to answer this question. But while considering my family's story and the hundreds of other families' stories, my answer kept coming back as "It depends on what is happening in your life." In other words, the starting point can and will be different depending on your unique circumstances. The big picture is more like a circle of responsibilities. Enter and exit as needed.

"Making a Plan" addresses the essential of who should do what and when. Having a plan is so much better than not having a plan. Different personalities have different strengths and different weaknesses. If possible, examine these differences and assign duties to those most able. If doing it alone, manage your time wisely.

Worrying about money is also a good place to start, so "Collecting Essential Paperwork" is for the family member who knows the legal and financial industries. This person will know to be diligent with all the specific details these industries require. If you don't know what I mean, be sure to read the section on how to title bank and brokerage accounts.

The essential of "Taking Care of the Person" is deliberately titled. Being sensitive to the whole person is critical as we introduce what changes to expect and to accept. Physical and mental abilities are diminishing, but the essence of who they are remains. Nursing skills come into play for this section. Medical help is great, but knowing what can be expected will ease concerns. Ideas on what to do while maintaining respect help to keep you aware in a loving way. My thoughts turn to the wife who constantly assured her husband that his forgetfulness was a result of his recent surgery. She was taking care of a very important person in her life.

In working with my seniors, my staff and I learned to see them as valuable members of society. Each individual had a story to tell, and we were ready and excited to listen. I so wish I were better at "Recording the Legacy" for all of my seniors. I've tried to relate some stories for this essential. How I wish I had written these stories as they were spoken. Please make time now for your family stories.

"Choosing a New Home" is a great group activity for any family. It can be such an easy step in the natural progression of life. Think about whether it would be more fun to visit your loved one where they live currently or where they might live in the future. Also, consider the option of home modifications. There is no one answer that fits all, which is why there are so many options.

The example of a typical senior move can illustrate how these five essentials come into play. When a family member contacted me about moving, I knew that they had already chosen a new home. The community required copies of POAs and DNRs, so collecting essential paperwork had to be done ahead of time. While evaluating how and when to move, the family would let us know of any physical or emotional issues. The need to have the bed ready for an afternoon nap often had to be part of our plan. Their family plan made sure that there was one family member who would be our contact person for the move. And listening to the stories, as I said earlier, made every move a joy.

As one of my sisters said, "You've taken a maze and turned it into a straight line." I hope you, the reader, experience this same clarity as you explore the five essentials.

CHAPTER 3

MAKING A PLAN

Building on what we've learned so far, we should be ready to make a plan. The team is ready. The senior is ready. So let's discuss some plan options.

The "Long-Term" plan is a best solution. It's the gradual approach my family used. The "Middle Ground" plan assumes a tighter time schedule of, say, five or fewer years. I hope you can avoid the "Need to Do It Now" plan, but having a plan is better than no plan at all.

All of these plans can work. Over the course of the next few chapters, differences will be pointed out; the tools presented are pretty much the same for all of these plans. The main differences are time and control. Hold the image of your special person in your mind's eye as we discuss making a plan.

WHEN YOU HAVE LOTS OF TIME

The "Long-Term" plan is the best solution because it's the gradual approach. Time and control are pretty flexible. All team members are actively engaged in a slow, steady acceptance of end-of-life issues. Life-affirming tasks, such as storytelling, can be given a lot of time. Control mainly rests with the senior; the team can focus on accountability by completing the "Master Checklist."

WHEN YOU HAVE LESS THAN FIVE YEARS

The "Middle Ground" plan assumes a tighter time schedule of less than five years. A perfect example is the annual visit to your grandparents. Somehow the house seems more dusty than usual. A check of the refrigerator shows some food should be thrown out and the pantry also has some expired food (most pantries do, so you can make a joke about this). Generally, the awareness of aging has risen to a level of concern. Time and control are still on your side at this point. Accountability and measurable results are more insistent. You need to complete that "Master Checklist."

WHEN YOU HAVE NO TIME

The "Need to Do It Now" plan is for situations with no time, no control. Well, not exactly, but that is how everyone will feel because the doctor is now in control. The team has to act immediately. The loved one needs help right away. It's an emergency, so everyone will do everything possible to adjust to these circumstances. Making this plan work will be discussed next, with ideas and hints about bringing control back to the team.

Whatever the time frame for your plan, congratulations. You're on the way to being decisive about the future and how it might unfold. Personal considerations will take priority. The family team approach to a plan for aging graciously is taking shape.

MASTER CHECKLIST WITH TIME CONSIDERATION

Do It Now

- CHOICES FOR REHAB (3)

- CHOICES FOR HOME CARE (3)

- CLEANING PERSON: REGULAR

- ESTATE ATTORNEY

- CERTIFIED PUBLIC ACCOUNTANT (CPA)

- HEALTH COMPANION

Sooner Rather than Later

- SENIOR MOVE MANAGER

- CHOICES FOR SENIOR LIVING COMMUNITIES (3)

- REALTOR

- GUN SELLER

- JEWELRY BUYER

- COINS/PRECIOUS METALS BUYER

- FUNERAL DIRECTOR

- SHREDDING SERVICE

Later

- CLEANING PERSON: DEEP CLEANING

- APPRAISER

- AUCTION HOUSE

- ESTATE SALES COMPANY

- DONATION PICKUP

- JUNK REMOVAL

NEED TO DO IT NOW PLAN

The doctor is in control for now. Something serious has occurred, and this is now an emergency situation.

The Doctor-Patient Perspective

After evaluating the patient, the medical team has determined that further assistance is required. When it's time to leave the hospital, this additional assistance will need to be ongoing. Upon release from the hospital, someone will need to take charge of this person's care.

Can the person holding the MD POA be present for doctor/patient conversations? Most of us without medical experience are in unfamiliar territory. Level of care issues will be discussed. Learning to navigate this world of strange terminology is hard, but not impossible.

Control will be turned over to the team very shortly. Take control by having the designated health companion present for every conversation with the doctor. This companion accompanies a patient on all doctor or medical appointments. Since we all hear and remember conversations differently, this extra set of ears can be a real comfort. (Recording these conversations or using FaceTime communications are also acceptable options.)

REHAB CENTER ISSUES

The doctor says that your loved one will need extensive rehabilitation (for example, after a stroke or broken hip). A social worker team may be assigned to help the family. This hospital team will likely suggest a rehab center that has an opening. Extensive rehab sets off alarms in my head, which is why its discussion rates a separate section on "Rehab Concerns" later in this chapter.

You can control the level of care equation. If a rehab center is recommended, know that you have the ability to go to one you have chosen—space available, of course. If an assisted living community is one of the options presented, then the decision on at least three possible "new homes" can be revisited.

First impressions are good indicators for these choices. What names of communities come to mind? If you've made the team and had the conversation, you are ready with answers. If you haven't, then someone can be tasked to make these calls or visits. Decisions on the size will be required, as well as cost. Again, space availability will be a consideration.

In "Need To Do It Now" situations, my strong advice is to contact a Senior Move Manager® (SMM). This industry has been around since before 2005. I didn't start there, but it is where I acquired a lot of education on issues of aging. The National Association of Senior Move Managers (NASMM) can locate a SMM for you. Go to their website (nasmm.org) for all kinds of suggestions.

Decisions have had to be made quickly. The emergency has been handled, and getting this loved one to the next safe place is happening.

ACTIVITIES OF DAILY LIVING (ADL)

These self-care tasks vary from five to fourteen depending on whom you ask. A person needs assistance with two to six to activate a long-term care insurance policy.

- BATHING AND GROOMING (BATHING)

- DRESSING AND UNDRESSING (DRESSING)

- MEAL PREPARATION AND FEEDING (EATING)

- FUNCTIONAL TRANSFERS (GETTING IN AND OUT OF BED)

- SAFE RESTROOM USE AND MAINTAINING CONTINENCE (TOILETING)

- AMBULATION (WALKING, GETTING OUTSIDE)

- MEMORY CARE AND STIMULATION (ALZHEIMER'S DISEASE AND DEMENTIA)

INSTRUMENTAL ACTIVITIES OF DAILY LIVING (IADL)

IADLs allow a person to function independently in a community.

- TAKING MEDICATIONS CORRECTLY

- USING THE PHONE

- GROCERY SHOPPING

- PREPARING MEALS

- HOUSEKEEPING

- LAUNDERING

- USING TRANSPORTATION

- MANAGING FINANCES

NEED TO DO IT NOW PLAN

What? I can't go home? How did this happen? I don't know where I am, but I am OK … I think. The doctor has done all his testing. He says I can't go home.

The doctor is in control. Welcome to the worst case scenario as far as the senior is concerned.

THE SENIOR PERSPECTIVE

I'm so afraid!

The doctor says I can't go home. I need more help. OK. My team has come to terms with that option. But I can't stay here either. What to do? If I need help, can't I get help at home? I always thought I'd die in my own bed. What to do? Several of my friends have moved into that new independent living community out East. Should I go join them? And is that even an option, since the doctor says I need help? What to do? And I need to do it soon.

A good first step is having someone with you whenever there is information passed along, so choose a health companion, your partner in listening carefully. Pick a good listener from your community of family and friends. Either you or this health companion should be able to ask questions—the right questions.

The number one question is always, When can I go home? But this is not necessarily the right question. The first question should be, What do I have to do to be able to go home? This implies a team approach to getting well.

What is the question uppermost in your mind after hearing that someone is in the hospital? Is this person OK? First you have to be OK. Go with this thought. You'll hear me repeat this a lot. Take care of yourself first. You have to be OK to go home.

If you've had "The Senior Conversation" with your family, then you might have a team with the beginnings of a plan. At least you've talked about it. The question now is how to take control quickly. It's time to enjoy the privilege of accepting help.

Who is going to make me comfortable, while I try to get well? What happens if the doctor says I can't go home?

Understanding where you are in life's journey is harder for some than for others. I know of one woman who listened carefully to her prognosis after a serious fall. Considering her options, she talked to her spiritual advisor. She chose to refuse food from that point on. The day before her fall had been one of the best days of her life, so she was happy with this choice. What choice will you make?

But the doctor says that mobility will improve over time. How good is that!

It's going to take longer because the aging body takes longer. Don't panic. Be ready for the next step whatever that may be.

But the doctor says that from now on, I'll need daily help of some kind.

All these "buts" are saying you need to be more accepting of the current conditions. You know you need to concentrate on getting healthy.

You know you need to concentrate on returning yourself to where you were before all this happened. This is how to age gracefully.

SUGGESTED QUESTIONS FOR DOCTOR

Team's Thoughts and Questions

- IS GOING HOME A GOOD OPTION?

- WHEN DO YOU EXPECT (NAME) TO BE RELEASED FROM THE HOSPITAL, REHAB CENTER, ETC.?

- CAN I GET A FEW DAYS' PRIOR NOTICE SO I CAN PLAN MY SCHEDULE?

- WOULD YOU USE THIS REHAB CENTER FOR YOUR FAMILY MEMBER?

- CAN I GET A LIST OF AT LEAST THREE REHAB CENTERS SO I CAN CHECK THEM OUT MYSELF?

- IS DRIVING AN OPTION? WILL IT BE AN OPTION, GIVEN TIME? CAN YOU PUT THAT IN WRITING?

- CAN I BE TRAINED TO HANDLE WOUND CARE, ETC., ON MY OWN?

- CAN I GET A LIST OF AT LEAST THREE MEDICAL HOME CARE COMPANIES SO I CAN CHECK THEM OUT MYSELF?

Senior's Thoughts and Questions

* WHY CAN'T I GO HOME?

* WHAT DO I HAVE TO DO TO GET BETTER?

* WHAT DO I HAVE TO DO TO BE ABLE TO GO HOME?

* SHOULD I LOOK FOR INDEPENDENT OR ASSISTED LIVING?

* CAN I PLEASE HAVE A FAMILY MEMBER PRESENT TO HELP ME UNDERSTAND MY OPTIONS?

* CAN I PLEASE HAVE A FAMILY MEMBER HERE BEFORE WE TALK? I NEED SOMEONE TO LISTEN FOR ME.

NEED TO DO IT NOW PLAN

The doctor is in control for now.

The Team Perspective

How soon is soon? What is the best way for the team to help with this emergency? (For those of you who live out of town, time is a super-important consideration.) How long will it take you to get there? How much time will you need to take off work? How much longer will your loved one be staying in that place? And how much time does the family team have to make all these decisions? Answer: Don't panic. Take control.

Controlling decisions is what is required now. One decision at a time. Does anyone need to get there immediately? No. Your loved one is being cared for by professionals for the time being. Someone needs to listen to the doctor and the staff person, and most important, your senior loved one.

Communication

"Listen" is the operative word now. Quality listening is a unique skill. Prepare for the phone calls carefully. Make a list before the phone call; make another list after the phone call. Set up a conference call (pretty easy in today's world) with concerned family members so everyone gets the same information at the same time. Make another list. Communication is critical; informed communication is even better.

One question should be, "When is the expected release date?" In business terms, think of it as, "When is the project due?" My meaning here is to convert your desire to help into a manageable plan. Put your emotions and panic into a quieter place. "We'll get through this together" is what you want to communicate and what you should believe. Everyone needs gentle reassurances. Tell your loved one, "We'll do everything we can to make what you want happen."

Ask if you can schedule the release date for a Monday, Tuesday, Wednesday, or Thursday. Yes, you want to avoid the weekend, but this terminology is a better way of saying it. Why not the weekend? Because all the self-movers are occupying elevators on those days. You're more than that because you're a planner and a manager. You don't want your family exposed to this panic mode if at all possible.

Here's an example of a possible scenario. The Care Meeting was today, and the hospital wants to release your mom tomorrow, which is Friday. Her new room is being recarpeted and it won't be ready until Monday. And this weekend is the state tournament. Why does everything have to happen at once? The answer: it doesn't. Ask if it would be possible to move the release date to Monday. Ask your mom if that's OK first. Communicate your worries and concerns gently. You can tell her, "I know you want to get out of here, but it's the state tournament. I know you're safe here, so I won't worry about you this weekend. And the new place is great, but I want to be able to spend more time with you the first few days after the move. Is that OK?" Listen to her "true" answer; think about your "true" feelings. Decide.

Taking care of someone you love is hard, especially during an emergency. To be at your best, you have to take care of yourself as well. Follow these suggestions. Control is being passed to the team. You've got this.

Yeah, Team!

MOVING STEPS FOR ASSISTED LIVING WITH A SENIOR MOVE MANAGER

* WHEN IS THE EXPECTED RELEASE DATE?

* DECIDE ON LOCATION.

* HIRE A SENIOR MOVE MANAGER.

MOVING STEPS FOR ASSISTED LIVING WITHOUT A SENIOR MOVE MANAGER

- WHEN IS EXPECTED RELEASE DATE?

- DECIDE ON LOCATION.

- GET A FLOORPLAN.

- CREATE A DETAILED FURNITURE LAYOUT.

- MARK FURNITURE.

- DECIDE ON DATE OF MOVE.

- HIRE MOVING COMPANY.

- PACK, WITH UNPACKING IN MIND.

- MAKE THE NEW PLACE FEEL JUST LIKE HOME.

CONTACTS FOR MOVE

NAME

MOVING FROM: **OLD ADDRESS**

MOVING TO: **NEW ADDRESS**

	STREET	CITY	ZIP CODE
OLD ADDRESS			
NEW ADDRESS			

CONTACTS ORIGIN

COMPANY/CONTACT NAME	PHONE	MOBILE	E-MAIL
FAMILY/FRIEND			
MOVE MANAGER			
MOVER			
DRIVER			

CONTACTS DESTINATION

COMPANY/CONTACT NAME	PHONE	MOBILE	E-MAIL
FAMILY/FRIEND			
MOVE MANAGER			
MOVER			

REHAB CONCERNS

What if you've never had to rehab? What if, at an advanced age, you are suddenly told you will need to spend some time in a rehab center?

If one has ever had to rehab from an injury or a surgery, you know the drill. Wait for the prescribed amount of time to heal. Begin the journey back to health. Accept the "new normal."

If you have ever played any sport, it is likely that you have experienced this same range of instructions. If you have needed to rehab before, you are at an advantage. You already understand the need to wait. ("Waiting is." *Stranger In A Strange Land* by Robert A. Heinlein.) And the need to perform a set or sets of exercises is also a recognized step in the healing process. The "new normal" is the final stage. You can do everything again, but now you have a scar if you have had surgery. You can do everything again, but only after stretching or warming up slowly if you have had muscle strains or sprains. You can do everything again, but have a fear of falling if you have broken a bone. These are real-life examples.

Reevaluate the Master Checklist

What does the team think? In many ways, rehab time is an excellent time to reevaluate your "Master Checklist." Home care choices are very likely in the near future. Even if you're hiring someone for only two hours a day, home care agencies or individuals can be tested on response time, personality, and ability to understand and deal with the conditions your loved one is experiencing. Compatibility with family members can also be addressed.

A cleaning person might be found who specializes in circumstances like your current one. If your loved one left home in an ambulance, the home may have been left in disarray. The family might have had time to clean up. Friends and neighbors often pitch in. Cleaning services bring all the necessary equipment and supplies, then make things tidy and smelling fresh in a short amount of time. Generally, the company I recommended accomplished this feat in two hours or less. How much is your time worth?

The health companion is on alert during this time. If possible, provide breaks for this person. Take care of the health companion as much as you are taking care of the injured person. This role comes with a set of hard-to-define emotions. During the "break," take the time to listen to these feelings. Such consideration will be a special step in uniting the family team.

Evaluate the Rehab Center

Evaluating the rehab center in real time is another imperative. Stop in at different times, and start a mental checklist. Be aware of how much time your rehabbing senior spends in their room versus how much time is spent in the common areas. Time spent in bed should also be on your radar, as this is when pressure sores occur. Eating issues may develop, so take some time to eat together. Try the food your loved one is served, but try to provide favorite meals as well. Broasted chicken, shrimp salad sandwiches, and raw oysters were my mom's favorites, so the hour it took her to consume them was time well spent.

CAUTION

Know that horror stories about rehab centers are real. This is the one situation in which I encourage you to worry. Special care of a loved one is critical for the team. Daily visits are a must. Do not relax this behavior until the more permanent location is attained.

Rehab time puts so many things in perspective. It forces each member of the family team to recognize where you are on this journey of aging. Make peace with each other. Accept and refine your role in the process.

THE MIDDLE GROUND PLAN

The team is in control. The team includes the senior.

A much better plan than the "Need To Do It Now" plan is the middle-ground approach. In my Introduction to this book, you met two ladies who used this solution. Basically, the plan is to give you a set amount of time to be ready to move. The good part is now you are totally in control. And control is a much better solution.

Let's go back to the example of the annual, often holiday, visit to a grandparent. This example was chosen because it happened so often in my SMM business. Generally, awareness of aging has risen to a level of concern. This new awareness that it's time to do something, before things get worse, is the catalyst. It makes having the senior conversation more important, but so much easier than if it had been an internal trigger. Dust and expired food can be dealt with gently. "Tell us what you want and we'll do everything we can to make it happen," with the one caveat of a time limit.

Coming to a Consensus

Initially, the option of staying home should be part of the discussion. Ask, "What does that look like? Are you safe? Can you take care of yourself?" The answers to these questions should come from the senior. Then the answers should come from you. Remember, building a consensus is the beginning of a real plan. The question of safety is paramount. This question needs to be asked and answered by all parties to all parties' satisfaction. The team can then move forward together.

Employing Outside Help

Employing outside help can be a comfortable option. For families who live out of town, or for families without the patience or time, outside professional help can be the answer. Outside help comes in many forms. Initially, home care can be as infrequent as two hours per day. Regular cleaning can be once a month. Trusted caregivers can also be a comfort in these situations. Your team decides.

Valuables

A major concern when employing outside help is fear of theft, a common complaint in the senior community. Although it happens infrequently, the fear is always there. The easiest way to avoid this concern is to remove all financial records, jewelry, and other expensive items to a safe location prior to contacting an organizer, a move manager, or a caregiver for help. A virtual inventory is always a great idea. Pictures of valuables, along with an estimate of replacement costs, can be used as proof for insurance or police reports. Official appraisals bring comfort to some families. Whatever your method, make a written list of which family members get specific items.

What about the "stuff"? Become comfortable with my F.A.S.T. (Family, Argh, Sell, Trash) approach. By employing this method of sorting, you'll learn that the good family treasures and the not-so-good trash items are easily distinguishable. The Sell or Argh (Donate) items can take up as much time as you want. Consider this statement: The most valuable asset most people own is their house. Don't let the stuff distract you. Take care of value first.

HOW TO SORT F. A. S. T.

Where do I start? Organizing for your move can be done both prior to and/or after your move.

1.   CHOOSE AN EASY TASK.

2.   SET A TIMER.

3. USE FOUR CORNERS OF ROOM FOR SELECTION, THEN USE THREE-SECOND DECISION TIME.

4. EXAMINE WHAT YOU'VE DONE. (YOU CAN RE-SORT AS MANY TIMES AS YOU LIKE, BUT ...)

5. FINISH WHAT YOU START.

Family

*   JEWELRY

*   PHOTOS

*   IMPORTANT PAPERS

*   JUST BECAUSE

Argh!

*   GENTLY USED CLOTHING

*   POTS/PANS/DISHES

*   EXTRA OFFICE SUPPLIES

*   BOOKS

Sell

*   OLD TOYS

- ANY CERAMIC ITEM WITH A MARKING

- ANYTHING UNUSUAL/HISTORICAL

- A "WHAT IS IT?"

Trash

- WORN-OUT SHOES/BOOTS

- RUSTY POTS/PANS

- BROKEN LAMPS

THE LONG-TERM PLAN

The team is in control. The team includes the senior.

External triggers remind you that there's no time like the present to formulate a long-term plan. How many times have you heard someone say, "I'm going to take care of things now so my kids don't have to go through this"? Usually, these thoughts consume a person after attending a funeral. And the age of seventy-five should put everyone on alert. Even extremely healthy seventy-five-year-olds should have a medical POA (also known as an *advance directive*). Preparing an actionable plan is where we're headed.

A good example is the plan proposed by my son-in-law's grandfather. My understanding is that the family had a brief "conversation" about the grandmother. She moved on to a life in memory care; her husband died shortly after. And the family closed the chapter on the place where they grew up. Do you recognize this scenario? Can you relate?

Since this is a long-term plan, think of your tasks as continuing short-term goals. Staying at home, with outside help, was discussed in the "Middle Ground" plan and applies here as well. Staying at home, by way of home modifications, is another good option. Relocating the bedroom to the main level, installing a stair elevator, and building an entrance ramp are home modifications easily available to the general public. These tasks ensure both the senior and the team are comfortable.

Storytelling and going over old photos are some other tasks that provide comfort. And they also make the process fun. Use this time to retell and possibly record old family stories. But don't put off the accountability task. Begin looking at the "Master Checklist with Timelines," which you learned about earlier in this chapter. You'll need to complete this in the next chapter.

Dealing with Possessions

Now that the team, including the senior member, is comfortable, it's time to talk about the "stuff." Getting rid of things will make you feel better. It has measurable rewards for everyone. Try my F.A.S.T. method—it's the method we used in my SMM company when called upon to empty a house so it could be sold. I know it works because I had to do this for an average of fifty families every year for eleven years.

What makes the F.A.S.T. method work even better is creating a simple spreadsheet of the house. As part of your long-term plan, you're going to come up with a way to "see" all those hidden places where things seem to have a life of their own. The spreadsheet layout will help you stay on task, room by room. It's also a concrete piece that everyone can go back to in order to see what has been accomplished. I'm a big fan of celebrating successes with aging people. (Actually, with anyone.) But a spreadsheet is also a tool that can show measurable results. In case something changes suddenly, you will already have a tool to speed up the timeline. Control, success, celebration; all this is definitely possible.

A related important task is making a list of who gets what. Included on this list would be jewelry, firearms, artworks, and other expensive items that should be handled differently and carefully (before hiring outside help). And there are always family "treasures" whose value is known and measured only by family members.

HOUSE ROOM LOCATOR

Below is a chart that will help you get a complete count of the number of rooms, shelves, and cabinets, so you can get an estimate of the amount of time needed to clear away all items. Assume at least an hour for each room, but add more time, depending on the level of density. (I used full, half-full, and easy for my estimates.) Revise room names as needed.

HOUSE ROOM LOCATOR

UPPER LEVEL

HALL	SITTING AREA	MASTER	MASTER CLOSET	PATIO	BEDROOM 2	LINEN

SHELVES/ CABINETS
DENSITY ESTIMATE
TIME ESTIMATE
OTHER COMMENTS

MAIN LEVEL

DINING	OFFICE	LIVING	KITCHEN	PATIO	LAUNDRY	GARAGE

SHELVES/CABINETS
DENSITY ESTIMATE
TIME ESTIMATE
OTHER COMMENTS

LOWER LEVEL

HALL	STORAGE 1	BEDROOM	LIVING	POOL ROOM	BAR	STORAGE 2

SHELVES/CABINETS
DENSITY ESTIMATE
TIME ESTIMATE
OTHER COMMENTS

OUTSIDE

FRONT	SHED	

SHELVES/CABINETS
DENSITY ESTIMATE
TIME ESTIMATE
OTHER COMMENTS

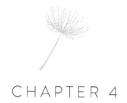

CHAPTER 4

CHOOSING A
NEW HOME

B ased on the doctor's advice and discussions with your loved one, it may be time to choose a new home. As with most decisions, there are several options available to you, and some new terminology will be attached.

Which type of community is the right one for your loved one? The three main types are independent living (IL), assisted living (AL), and skilled nursing (SNF, pronounced *ska-niff*). Before I describe these options, one more acronym should be introduced. Continuing care retirement communities (CCRC) offer the option of taking you from your current needs to the end of life. In other words, they include IL, AL and SNF services at, basically, the same location.

A memory care residence is another type of community which your doctor may decide is needed; hospice and palliative care is a living arrangement which will also be discussed at the end of this section.

INDEPENDENT LIVING

Independent living (IL) is the most desirable option for those who are still quite capable. IL communities provide meals in a dining room, an exercise room onsite, and transportation to shopping, outside events, medical appointments, and a variety of other needs. Giving up cooking is a comfort for many who choose this lifestyle. Experiencing a social network of peers is one of the best things I have seen at this type of community. Playing bridge, shooting pool, and playing bingo are games that residents seem to enjoy. An activity director generally provides something different to do each day.

ASSISTED LIVING

Assisted living (AL) provides a higher level of care because it's needed. More new terminology: AL seniors need more help with activities of daily living (ADLs). Getting dressed, taking proper medications, and toileting are primary examples of ADLs. You might be able to handle these issues for your loved one, but moving your loved one to an AL community is a good option. You'll know when it's time.

Some advice: Seniors who resist relocating to AL can be allowed to go to IL for a trial period. When getting someone to a safe place, that is, out of their home, is the primary consideration, using the logic of a trial period in IL can ease disagreement and provide a middle-ground option.

SKILLED NURSING

Skilled nursing (SNF) is the option dreaded by so many seniors. "Don't put me in the nursing home! I'm not ready to die!" might be your loved one's first reaction. Fear is doing the talking now. Crying together can help, as can daily hugs. If at all possible, communicate that "we're going to get through this together somehow." Fear of abandonment also needs to be addressed. Make contact daily to alleviate this fear. Reminding yourself and your loved one that the old nursing home model no longer exists may help. Recovery from strokes and broken bones is more likely given modern medical advances. Reminding everyone that skilled nursing staff expect you to get better can also help.

MEMORY CARE

Memory care is another solution if forgetfulness has progressed to the point where it can be dangerous to leave your loved one alone. Forgetting the way home or forgetting that something is on the stove are examples of behaviors that require intervention. Those concerned individuals who see your loved one on a daily basis are often the first to recognize memory troubles. My mom always seemed fine to me, but my sister became seriously alarmed when sundowning had my mother cooking in the middle of the night. Also be aware that the anesthesia necessary for surgery can bring on temporary bouts of extreme forgetfulness.

Eventually, take advantage of memory care residences. You'll experience more sleep and more enjoyment of visits. Frequently, a senior will enjoy life more as well because of the structure provided in memory care.

HOSPICE AND PALLIATIVE CARE

When the doctor recommends hospice and palliative care know that the end can be a closer event. One choice for this type of care is to move to a room in a hospital, on a floor designated for hospice care. Often, the choice to remain at home is selected. One benefit of the hospital setting is the sense that you are leaving sorrow behind in that location. Decide what works best for your family.

MASTER LIST WITH ASSIGNMENTS

ACTIVITY	FAMILY MEMBER	START DATE
CHOICES FOR REHAB (3)		
CHOICES FOR HOME CARE (3)		
CLEANING PERSON: REGULAR		
ESTATE ATTORNEY		
FINANCIAL ADVISOR		
CPA		
HEALTH COMPANION		
CHOICES FOR SENIOR LIVING COMMUNITIES (3)		
SENIOR MOVE MANAGER		
REALTOR		
GUN SELLER		
JEWELRY BUYER		
COINS/PRECIOUS METALS BUYER		
FUNERAL DIRECTOR		
CLEANING PERSON: DEEP CLEANING		
APPRAISER		
AUCTION HOUSE		
ESTATE SALES COMPANY		
DONATION PICKUP		
JUNK REMOVAL		

COMMUNITY SELECTION

The decision to find a "new home" is now uppermost in the team's mind. Think of it as making a real estate purchase. You want to feel at home as soon as you walk in the door. Subconsciously, you check out the neighbors. Does this place require any maintenance on our part? What's the cost? And what's included in that cost? We really want a turnkey establishment.

Amenities vary from community to community, so visiting is highly recommended. Almost all community managers invite you to lunch. Often included at this meal are satisfied, friendly residents who can share their impressions of life at the community. Following (or preceding) lunch is a tour. Take mental pictures of the activities in the common rooms, where you should see residents doing what they do every day. Common areas are usually the library, the pool room, and the exercise room. Is there a community room with computers? Try to have a brochure from the community with you so you can take notes. Stay positive on this first visit. Comparing community amenities will tax your mental abilities unless your team has written comments.

On this first visit, ask about the activities director. Frequently, the community manager can provide a printed schedule of activities for you. A good activity director is very likely in a class; getting to watch him or her in action is a plus.

Getting to watch the rest of the staff in action is also a plus. The front desk receptionist/concierge needs to be gracious but firmly in control. The cleaning staff should be friendly but stay out of the way during your visit. (Take notes on how they treat the seniors.)

The maintenance staff were some of my favorites while I had my business. You *should* see them at work. In a community of fifty-plus rooms, there is always something that needs to be fixed or updated. Gracious, friendly, aware—these are the characteristics to look for in the staff.

Services can also fall under the category of amenities, but they are somewhat different. A hair salon onsite means getting pampered with hair and nail treatments is convenient . Doctors making resident calls is a fairly new and very welcome addition to services at some communities. A driver, who can be scheduled to take you to doctors' visits, can be a comfort. And the bus trips to the grocery stores are also a welcome service.

Make yourself a note to ask if there are guest rooms or respite rooms. Respite care, by definition, is short-term relief for primary caregivers. Guest rooms allow family members to stay onsite for their visits; respite rooms allow caregivers to get breaks, while elderly family members enjoy a change of environment. Obtaining this information during community visits is a good idea.

The overall size of the community is another aspect you might be concerned about. Senior living communities vary from as few as ten rooms to as many as four hundred rooms. Don't forget to ask how far it is to the dining room. While some residents might enjoy a long walk after dinner, some do not. In larger communities, residents actually drive to meals.

Location, location, location. Close to family would be my one stipulation. While social friends and church friends are important, family is first. Moving to be with family does make sense. And, if that means an out-of-state move, yes, it will be hard.

Visit at least three communities, with the same family member if at all possible. Together, the team can find the best "new home," a place to live for the remainder of the senior's days.

COMMUNITY CONSIDERATIONS

(print three copies so you can compare)

Activities

- EXERCISE

- COMPUTER USE

- CLASSES

- OUTSIDE ENTERTAINMENT

Transportation

- FOR DOCTOR'S APPOINTMENTS

- FOR GROCERY SHOPPING

Amenities

- POOL

- MOVIE THEATER

- HAIR SALON

- LAUNDRY

- LIBRARY

- POOL ROOM

- GUEST ROOMS/RESPITE ROOMS

Dining

- FOOD QUALITY

- CLEANLINESS

- COMFORT

APARTMENT SELECTION

Choosing an apartment within a community can be as simple as looking at floorplans online. For those of us who need to see and feel our surroundings, it's time to take a tour. Most communities offer scheduled tours of their different apartments. Often, these apartments have been staged to give a better idea of just how comfortable any size apartment can be, given the right amount and size of furniture. Sometimes, community managers ask residents to show off their living arrangements. All of these instances provide visual ideas and expectations. The perfect solution to relocating is almost here.

Begin by examining your current living situation. Where do you spend most of your time? The bedroom, of course, because eight hours of sleep is the norm. After that, how much time is spent reading, watching TV, and cooking? Which room or rooms are you using now? Frequently, the living room is the main room for reading and TV enjoyment. Those who use computers might have a desk in the kitchen, living room, or a separate room. And how much cooking will happen when meals are provided as part of your monthly cost? Determining which rooms are used on a daily basis is an easy task for senior move managers, who do these evaluations on a regular basis. For example, formal dining rooms are becoming a thing of the past. Answering the questions on this page will help you choose the right size apartment.

Size

How big is big enough? Older couples often choose a two-bedroom apartment, but one-bedroom apartments are the most common choice. What size seemed best when your team visits? Apartment sizes vary, as do individual rooms, so take some time to get the size right. A search of several community websites showed the following:

IL (Independent Living)
436 sq. ft. studio to 1520 sq. ft. garden home

AL (Assisted Living)
364 sq. ft. studio to 1144 sq. ft. 2 bedroom

SNF (Skilled Nursing Facility)
320 sq. ft. to 535 sq. ft. private and semi-private

Memory care
320–535 sq. ft. private and semi-private

Location

Unit size isn't your only consideration. What about neighbors? Do you want someone living above you? After all, this is an apartment building, so neighbor issues need to be addressed. How loud is the noise from the next-door neighbor? Can you hear the next-door neighbor or their pet? What are the rules regarding pets? Location of the apartment should also be considered. How close do you want to be to the laundry room or elevator? (And the conversations held there?) How close to the dining room would be optimal for you? Consider all of these questions before deciding.

Cost

Cost, however, may be the determining factor. Try to be realistic about how much can be spent on a monthly basis. Give yourself a range of numbers to play with. Retirement communities are more often run by larger corporations that demand a certain rate of return. Depending on which state you live in, costs will vary widely.

For example, an internet search in 2019 delivered the news that fifteen hundred to six thousand dollars per month can be expected. And don't forget that an annual increase is not unusual. Find out before signing any contracts.

Furniture Layout

Visualizing the new furniture layout is a good strategy when trying to make the new living situation feel "just like home." After creating a detailed measurement of the new apartment, place it onto a magnetic space-planning board. This tool allows all interested parties to move furniture pieces around the new room. Eventually, agreement on what will fit and what won't fit will result. (Please note: Coffee tables eat up a lot of space and are tripping hazards.)

Your goal: Choose the right size apartment and the right amount of furniture in the right location.

CHOOSING THE RIGHT APARTMENT

Cost

- MONTHLY

- EXTRAS

Size

(floor planning is important)

- MAGNETIC SPACE-PLANNING BOARD

- FLOORPLAN SOFTWARE

Location

- TOP FLOOR

- GROUND FLOOR (THOSE WITH PETS)

- CLOSE TO:

  - DINING ROOM

  - ELEVATOR

  - LAUNDRY

  - ACTIVITIES

MEMORY CARE

Memory issues deserve their own discussion. Dementia is a general term for the changes that cause memory loss in the aging brain. Parkinson's disease is one form of dementia. And we are all familiar with the diagnosis of Alzheimer's disease. *Still Alice* by Lisa Genova is a great book to read (or movie to watch) to familiarize yourself with this memory-stealing disease. Unreasonable anger is one of the major warning signs. Often, when people realize their memory is failing, it makes them resentful. When you are confronted by unreasonable anger in a senior friend or relative, it is wise to consider whether it might be because they inherently realize they are losing precious thoughts.

Personal experience seems to be the best way to consider this topic. My younger sister noticed that my mother's conversations were becoming repetitive. As her concern grew, I began calling more often to verify her observations. I wasn't sure if I wanted to agree or disagree with her take on the situation. My mother was always "up" for our conversations. (I live halfway across the country while my mother was on the East Coast.) She asked about the kids, remembered their names, and wanted to know how my husband was liking his work. All in all, a normal, congenial conversation. What was my sister talking about?

My next in-person visit made me aware that dementia is not a constant—at least in my mother's case. My quarterly visit, designed to give my sister a break as well as to spend time with Mother, brought the memory problems into focus. Simple conversations seemed the most difficult for Mother to remember.

"Where are we going?" Mother would ask. "Oh, yeah." "We did that yesterday? Oh, yeah."

Her short-term memory was abandoning her. After several days of repeated questions and the same answers, I understood my sister's point; something was definitely going on in my mother's brain.

While visiting, I was able to observe one of the memory tests given by her doctor. Mother was asked to count backward, what day of the week it was, and who was president. She had perfect answers for all of these questions. At the beginning of the session she was asked to remember three words or pictures. At the end of the session she was asked what those three things were. I think she remembered one. Memory issues diagnosed.

As short-term memory fades, access to long-term memories can become clearer. One time, my mother began talking about how much fun we had taking the ferry to the beach. She chatted on for a while about that day. It was obviously a lovely memory. When she finally looked up, she said, "Oh, you're not ..." A sad and poignant moment for both of us. Sad that the story had to end. Sad that I couldn't be that person for just a little while longer.

If you would like to learn more about dementia, I suggest you embrace the opportunity to hear Teepa Snow (Look her up on You-Tube.) give a presentation on Alzheimer's. After showing you photos of how your brain starts to look like Swiss cheese, she slips into the persona of an Alzheimer's patient. It's a very real, in-your-face drama-tization—unforgettable, even as I sit here typing away.

Memory Care Residence Expectations

- ROOMS ARE VERY SMALL (320 TO 535 SQ. FT.)

- NEED CODE FOR ENTRY AND EXIT (BE SURE DOOR CLOSES SECURELY)

- ENCLOSED OUTDOOR AREAS ARE SOMETIMES AVAILABLE

- RESIDENTS WANDER

- FINDING ANOTHER RESIDENT IN YOUR ROOM IS COMMON

- COMPLAINTS MAY OR MAY NOT BE TRUE

- SOME RESIDENTS ASK FOR HELP EVERY FEW MINUTES (OFTEN LOUDLY)

- DO NOT BRING ANY VALUABLES

- PUT NAME ON CLOTHING USING A PERMANENT MARKER

Residents like the structure of:

- FOLDING CLOTHES

- TAKING CARE OF BABY DOLLS

- DISCUSSING CURRENT EVENTS (NICE SURPRISE)

- PLAYING BINGO

- HAVING THE SAME TABLEMATES FOR MEALS

HOSPICE AND PALLIATIVE CARE

How many times have you heard the response, "I want to die at home"? What a great dream; dying on your own terms. Is it truly possible? With the help of those professionals trained in hospice and palliative care, the answer is a qualified yes. As I look back, I realize that at least four of my family members were helped to negotiate the end-of-life journey by theses angels of compassion. So what does hospice care look like?

Usually, one can rely on the doctor to make a judgment call about the timing for hospice to take over. You knew this time would arrive someday. It looks like your loved one's journey is coming to an end. The doctor, when asked, says it will be less than six months. Is acceptance of death something you can all agree on? It won't be easy. It hardly ever is. Let me introduce you to the concepts behind hospice (and palliative care).

Hospice Caregivers

The people who provide hospice care have responded and embraced a unique calling. Like those who work with cancer patients, they confront death on a daily basis and somehow make it OK. They are aware of the signs of impending death and they communicate with you about when to call in the family. If you haven't experienced an end-of-life situation yet, prepare to be amazed and welcomed.

People living their last days on earth are often aware that their days are numbered. Stories of last visits are numerous. A "rally" day can come when an out-of-state relative finally makes it in. So try to prepare, as much as humanly possible, to say goodbye. Prepare not so much for giving up the fight as for your loved one to say, "I'm ready to go. I'll miss you." And prepare your response.

Palliative Care

This is how everyone wants it to go. But what if severe pain is part of the equation? Palliative care is a fairly new way of saying that pain can be and needs to be managed aggressively. Opioids are often prescribed in these situations. The trick is to get the right dosage so your loved one can continue to communicate in as pain-free a manner as possible. Hospice workers take control in helping to determine the beneficial dosage. (And they often dispose of the unused medication in the proper manner.)

When my father passed away in the seventies, he had access to a "new" treatment at that time, using cocaine as the base for a pain reliever (the Brompton cocktail). All I can say is that we were all grateful that it gave him a way through his pain. He died at home encircled by family praying for him. More recently, my father-in-law and a brother-in-law also passed away at home while under the care of hospice professionals.

Dying at home is indeed possible.

PARTICIPATING IN THE ACTIVE DYING EXPERIENCE

Hearing is the last sense to go, so

- HAVE A LAST CONVERSATION

- HAVE MUSIC PLAYING SOFTLY

- SING; REMEMBER THOSE LULLABIES?

The sense of touch is the second-to-last sense to go, so

- HOLD HANDS

- USE GENTLE CARESSES

- GIVE KISSES

At the end:

- HOLD HANDS IN A CIRCLE AROUND THE PERSON LEAVING

- PRAY THE "LORD'S PRAYER" (OR YOUR PREFERRED PRAYER)

- SING

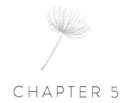

CHAPTER 5

TAKING CARE
OF THE PERSON

Taking care of the person requires that you see the person in a new light. Everyone has physical, mental, and emotional needs. As caregiving roles reverse and/or evolve, take time to consider what this role redefinition entails because now you are an actively involved decision helper. Your advice may or may not be used to make a decision.

Can you see why the senior conversation is so important? In the next few pages, I will discuss many of the ins and outs of taking care of an older adult. There are physical needs and emotional needs. There are legacy considerations and financial and legal concerns, which will be addressed in subsequent chapters.

RECOVERING FROM SURGERY

Some injuries caused by falls, car accidents, or other physical trauma can mean the body will heal only with surgical assistance. For example, hip fractures are more common in older people. Be aware that often the broken hip causes the fall, not the other way around. My point is that surgery can be a path to health. (A reminder: Anesthesia affects the brain of older adults more than expected. Be prepared for the brain fog, which may clear given enough time.) An example of the emotional reality for an actively involved decision helper follows.

The family shows outward calm, but of course there is inward turmoil. Your attention is geared toward your own concerns. This position is good and necessary; it's important to recognize your own feelings and deal with them.

Argh! The doctor wants to know who can make medical decisions if my loved one is incapacitated. Wasn't this supposed to be a routine hip replacement? This is so stressful!

But what about this person lying in bed in front of me? What should I be doing to make the thought of surgery less scary? What are our expectations for recovery?

Good for you! Your attention has turned to taking care of your loved one. Every attempt should be made to reassure the person going into surgery. Positive thinking often promotes positive results.

You are taking over your loved one's life. The need is confirmed. You can and will do this correctly. The team is as ready as it can be. Time to move ahead. Let's see where we stand on our "Master Checklist with Assignments." Yes, we are making progress.

MASTER LIST WITH ASSIGNMENTS - PROGRESS SO FAR

ACTIVITY	FAMILY MEMBER	START DATE	PROVIDER
HEALTH COMPANION			
CHOICES FOR REHAB (3)			
VISIT AND/OR INTERVIEW			
VISIT AND/OR INTERVIEW			
CHOICES FOR HOME CARE (3)			
VISIT AND/OR INTERVIEW			
VISIT AND/OR INTERVIEW			
CLEANING PERSON: REGULAR			
ESTATE ATTORNEY			
FINANCIAL ADVISOR			
CPA			

SENIOR LIVING COMMUNITIES			
VISIT AND/OR INTERVIEW			
VISIT AND/OR INTERVIEW			
SENIOR MOVE MANAGER			
REALTOR			
GUN SELLER			
JEWELRY BUYER			
COINS/PRECIOUS METALS			
FUNERAL DIRECTOR			

CLEANING PERSON: DEEP			
APPRAISER			
AUCTION HOUSE			
ESTATE SALES COMPANY			
DONATION PICKUP			
JUNK REMOVAL			

THE AGING BODY

The aging body gives many signals to let us know to be concerned about safety. There may be problems with eyes, ears, balance, bowels, incontinence, and memory—getting old is tough.

Eyes become cloudy from cataracts and macular degeneration; these eyes can't see the dust or the expiration dates on food or medicine. Ears gradually lose their ability to hear certain ranges of sound, so the TV is awfully loud. (Cautionary tale: When I spoke loudly to one of "my seniors," she told me she wasn't deaf, just old. Point taken.) Balance issues require removing throw rugs in the bathroom and any other tripping hazards. It's hard to discuss incontinence at any time, so be prepared with a small bag of extra clothing. Become aware of signals.

In my experience, it is fairly easy to divide these signals into what you see and what it takes a little more effort to notice. The senses of sight, smell, hearing, taste, and touch will serve as our guides for this discussion. The best way to stay on top of health issues is for the designated health companion to schedule and attend regular professional assessments of physical needs.

The gradual decline in the senses of sight and hearing are the most apparent and often go together. Successful movement requires seeing at the same time as hearing. Moving along on a city sidewalk or driving on a city street means these two senses are coordinated in processing the data being transmitted so that travel is efficient and safe.

Driving

Driving issues are probably the most difficult to confront. An older friend (eighty-five) recently insisted on driving us to the Chicago airport. *Oh my Gosh!* And you know what? It was great. She knew the city quite well, so after feeding us a traditional Hungarian meal in her apartment, she told us we would have to leave soon. She wanted to get back before dark, because she preferred driving during daylight hours. How perfect was that?

A different outcome can result if you don't confront the issue of driving in a timely manner. "Accidentally" running a red light can produce lifelong injuries for your loved one or for other persons involved in a car incident. Our great aunt now resides in assisted living because her car was in neutral rather than park. When she tried to stop the car from rolling down a hill, the car ran over her arm and broke her wrist. After several surgeries, she is lucky to be alive.

Have your loved one drive you somewhere so you can determine if the time to limit driving has arrived. Several states have restrictions for older adults to ensure safe driving, including yearly exams, no nighttime driving, or limited travel miles. These restrictions still allow for driving to the grocery store and the doctor. The ability to drive is a statement of freedom for most older adults.

In today's world, the option of using Uber or Lyft is a practical and almost perfect way of ending driving worries for all. It's even possible to purchase credits with these services, which can be gifted. Approach your driving questions practically as well as kindly, as often as needed.

Vision and Eye Health

What about healthy eyes and the sense of sight? Aging-eye issues include cataracts and macular degeneration. An eyechart taped to the bathroom mirror is a warning sign that the eye doctor is watching for macular degeneration. The diagnosis of cataracts can be met with calm as cataract surgery means the lens in the eye will be replaced. Some older adults even look forward to this diagnosis as it often means "No more losing your glasses." Any blurred vision is a warning sign. The ultimate solution is for the health companion to schedule and attend regular professional assessments of eye health.

Hearing

Effective hearing requires healthy ears. Hearing problems become apparent when conversations take unexpected turns: "Oh, I thought you said ..." The simplest solution is also the polite solution. When speaking to someone, make sure you look the person in the eye. This eye contact becomes the signal to listen and is a good life practice. If hearing still seems hard after employing this practice, it's time for a visit to the hearing specialist. Hearing aids are so small now that they are almost invisible. But they are also very expensive, so make sure there is a weighted container on the nightstand to protect this investment.

Other ear problems include wax buildup and vertigo. Wax buildup can be handled at home or in the doctor's office with lavage treatments. Vertigo upon standing is something you have probably experienced in your lifetime. Vertigo can also be a result of inner ear problems or medication issues. While hearing exams are not scheduled as regularly as other exams, the health companion should add this to the list of things to be monitored.

Taste and Smell

Let's now move the discussion to the gradual loss of the senses of taste and smell. Considering these two senses together is appropriate because that leads us to eating issues. When food doesn't taste as good as it used to, an older adult may not eat as much. Mealtime is a social function as well as a physical need. Eating with friends provides a nutritional and social benefit. The loss of the sense of smell also contributes to a lack of interest in food. Think of all the times you knew what your dinner was going to be just by the smell. Anticipation for the next meal is dulled when the sense of smell becomes muted. Memory of cooking smells can still get stomach juices flowing. It's time to make the effort to make eating more enjoyable. Weekly outings to a favorite restaurant can be a great solution for eating issues.

Dental Health

Dental health is also something to be discussed at this point. Your teeth do most of the work in chewing. It follows that your teeth need to be healthy. Dentures and implants address tooth loss. But mouth infections are very close to your brain. One friend, who had an abscessed tooth, learned that his infection came very close to killing him. An attentive friend insisted he see a dentist and therefore saved him. In some parts of the country, dental hygienists come to senior living communities to make it easier for seniors to maintain healthy teeth. Recently, in recognition of the importance of oral health, Medicare Advantage plans have added dental coverage. Verifying dental coverage and scheduling oral health visits adds one more item to our growing list of tasks for the health companion.

Touch

Personal hygiene, incontinence, and balance issues fall into the category of loss of sense of touch. Most obvious to me is the winter nose dripping. Little packets of Kleenex lovingly handed out as needed let your senior know that you respect and understand this loss of feeling in the nose. Loss of bowel sensations can lead to incontinence or constipation. Checking the underwear drawer gives you the ability to spot stubborn stains, which are your warning signs. Replacement underwear should be readily available as a nonconfrontational solution. Loss of bladder sensations can lead to urinary tract infections (UTIs), which are common among seniors. Drinking lots of water helps to solve dehydration problems as well as UTIs. Have your loved one drink from a large mug with measurements on the side to keep the knowledge of intake amounts in front of everyone. Just be aware, so you can keep the water container full.

One of my favorite client-provided solutions for some of the aging concerns discussed above is doing your loved one's laundry once a week. My client would schedule the weekly eating-out adventure for the same time. Easily planned and executed outings, with the added benefit of clothing oversight—and the pleasant smells of laundry handled by someone close to you—are pretty special.

FALL PREVENTION

The subject of balance and tripping also belongs in this category dealing with a diminished sense of touch. Combine slower reaction times with loss of feeling in your feet and you have a prescription for tripping and falling. Statistics from the National Institute on Aging remind us that 80 percent of falls happen in the bathroom. Placing rubber mats and/or shower seats in the tub area as well as installing side-of-the-tub grab bars are suggested by safety experts. Installing adjustable toilet seats with safety rails is an additional way to address fall prevention in the bathroom. I've spent a lot of time standing outside a bathroom door waiting in an "if-needed" mode. Privacy and safety are competing for your attention. They have equal weight at times, but the balance can seesaw at any time.

Other areas of the house should also be examined with the idea of fall prevention in mind. Removing throw rugs is a must. The beloved rocking chair is now a dangerous moving piece of furniture to be gifted appropriately. If newspapers and books are stacked on the floor beside a favorite chair, an end table will provide the better option. All chairs should have sturdy arms for help in rising from the seated position. These are all simple safety measures that provide comfort for all.

The last major concern is loss of memory, a special issue discussed previously in "Memory Issues."

Conclusion: Obviously, this is *not* a complete list of what can occur with your aging loved one. These examples are just some of the more common ones, and my purpose in presenting them has been to raise your awareness. These are some issues you need to become comfortable with if you are to be a caregiver for older family members or other seniors. Record what is "normal" for your individual and personal situation. Your planning is re-adjusting your lives gradually, and more important, your planning is avoiding a crisis.

One more thought: End-of-life issues are much like beginning-of-life issues. Keep this concept in mind as you review the next page.

HEALTH COMPANION TASKS

Schedule and attend:

PHYSICAL	ANNUALLY
VISION TEST	ANNUALLY
HEARING TEST	AS NEEDED
DENTIST VISIT	SEMI-ANNUALLY

OTHER FAMILY MEMBER TASKS

Schedule and attend:

EATING OUT	WEEKLY
HAIR STYLING	EVERY FOUR TO SIX WEEKS
NAIL APPOINTMENTS	EVERY FOUR TO SIX WEEKS

To be scheduled:

CLEANING SERVICE	SEMI-MONTHLY

REALITIES OF LIFE'S PROGRESSION

GROWING UP	GROWING OLD
SLEEP A LOT	SLEEP A LOT
WEAR DIAPERS	WEAR DIAPERS
WALK SLOWLY	WALK SLOWLY
NEED HELP WITH DRESSING	NEED HELP WITH DRESSING
NEED HELP WITH BATHING	NEED HELP WITH BATHING
NEED HELP WITH EATING	NEED HELP WITH EATING
TIRE EASILY	TIRE EASILY

***

THE EMOTIONAL ROLLER COASTER

For an older person, heading toward the end of life has many challenges. One of the most difficult to quantify is the emotional morass of isolation, loneliness, and a general feeling of being left out of the picture. It can be overwhelming unless the team takes a proactive approach.

As your loved one becomes increasingly frail, the desire to leave home seems to lessen. Going to the store or visiting friends becomes a challenge. Unknowingly, and perhaps, unwillingly, isolation sets in.

I used to resent my husband's weekly phone calls to his mom. Thinking about that now, I understand the joy those calls must have brought to her life. She had to give up driving. She had never developed a circle of friends. She enjoyed shopping, which had become her social outlet.

When you see a closet full of clothes with the price tags still on most of them, understand this: Shopping allows people to satisfy their need to be social. Having a salesperson see and talk to them satisfies their need for social interaction. As one client told me, she had to buy what the salesperson suggested, because that person had spent so much time helping her.

Loneliness is another word to describe this need for social interaction. Loneliness among older adults can be combatted with activities like bingo and card games like bridge and poker. Better still, since these diversions can be enjoyed at all ages, turn them into a family activity.

Venturing Out

I like to think I helped take care of my mom's emotional health with my quarterly visits. It was my way of replacing isolation or loneliness with adventure. Whenever I arrived at the house, she had her suitcase packed because she knew I was going to take her somewhere.

Although it's a major chore to take an older person out in public, the rewards are many. Did you know you can rent beach wheelchairs with large tires? Did you know that rooms for handicapped persons are perfect for giving older adults showers? I'm a big advocate of bringing older adults into the public eye as much as possible. Maybe wheelchair dancing at weddings will become a norm.

Feeling Left Out

Forgotten, But Not Gone: This is the original name I chose for my business helping seniors, but my friend's comment was, "You can't call it that. Too many seniors feel that way." (It was a play on words from the memorial page "Gone, But Not Forgotten" in the Air Force Academy magazine *Checkpoints*.) The perfect example was when I suggested an eighty-fifth birthday party for my mom, and she replied, "All my friends are dead." This feeling of being left out of the picture is sad, but true, and a very strong emotion for the living. Unless you make time to visit (one hour is the minimum amount of time, so plan accordingly), you may never understand this concept.

Fear

The final emotion I want to discuss is fear—fear of being taken advantage of, fear of falling, fear of growing old. Rational or irrational doesn't matter. Combat such fears simply by listening. We are walking this road together. Life has a beginning. Life has an ending. Fear becomes smaller with help. Emphasize again, we are here to help.

HELPING WITH NEGATIVE EMOTIONS: BE THERE

Dealing with Isolation

Get out on a regular basis

- MONTHLY INTEREST GROUP

- CRUISE

- BUS TRIP

- CHURCH

- FAVORITE RESTAURANT

- IN-PERSON VISIT

Dealing with Loneliness

All the above, plus the following:

- WEEKLY PHONE CALL

- EMAIL

- SOCIAL MEDIA (ONLY POSTINGS FROM FAMILY AND TRUE FRIENDS)

- PHOTO SHARING

Dealing with Fear

- SPEND THE NIGHT

- HOLD HANDS

- SHARE HUGS

- ABOVE ALL, LISTEN

CARE FOR THE CAREGIVER

Your days as an actively involved caregiver are beginning to feel endless. Stop right here! You are experiencing caregiver fatigue.

You're right. Somebody has to do it. But you don't have to be perfect. Setting limits is a necessary goal. Think of it this way: What would happen if you were suddenly incapacitated yourself? That's right. Someone else would have to make the decisions. Who should that someone be? A different family team member and/or a trusted individual are both good solutions. Taking care of yourself is so important; avoiding burnout is a necessity.

Family team members who live close by are overwhelmed more frequently than those who live out of town. Feelings of resentment can creep in. *How come I have to do it all?* Feelings of inadequacy begin to trouble your daily thoughts. *I don't know how much longer I can do this. These midnight phone calls are killing me.* So yes, you are going to take time off for rejuvenating and refocusing.

Different family team members should be recruited as part-time caregivers, on a planned schedule. Payment for family caregivers is entering the mainstream nowadays, so that's something to consider if one person assumes the majority of the responsibility.. My preplanned quarterly trips to help with my mom provided my sister with a known number of weeks to recuperate. Phone questions and updates brought the comfort of sharing feelings as well as ideas. Caregiving, with a live-in family member, is finally being recognized for what it is—a 24/7 commitment.

Solutions to caregiver fatigue are available. One of the better ones is *respite care*. Familiarize yourself with communities that provide this "short-term relief for primary caregivers." By using respite care for our mother, we discovered a memory care center that was the best one we had ever experienced. We were thankful she was able to stay there for the remaining years of her life.

Caregiver support groups also provide relief. Talking to someone going through similar trials is a comfort. Just being able to voice your feelings with someone who truly understands reaffirms the importance of your shared roles. Rejuvenate yourself by sharing your experiences and ideas.

Take time off so you can return with renewed energy.

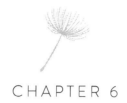

CHAPTER 6

COLLECTING ESSENTIAL PAPERWORK

Your loved one now needs you to address financial and legal concerns. Making a mental checklist, you're already wondering about the legal issues. Is there a will? If so, where is it? Are the bills getting paid? If they are, is this happening online or by mail? If it's online, is there a list of passwords? Is the password list safe? Yes, there are a lot of tasks to be accomplished.

It's time to get down to the bare bones of what the team needs to accomplish. We are going to begin with the *financial collection*, the *legal document collection*, and the *insurance collection*. I don't know if you remember, but *prepaid funeral services* were introduced in "Making the Team." Some of the terminology we'll discuss was also introduced in the beginning of the book.

TEAM INVENTORY

How has the inventory of your team's strengths and weaknesses progressed? Who is most suited to assume the financial role? Terms such as *individual retirement account* (IRA), *payable on death* (POD), and *trust* should be familiar to the designated person. *Do not resuscitate* (DNR) and *medical power of attorney* (MD POA) should be understood by the person willing to consider the physical ailments. (Thank goodness for the two nurses in my family.) Insurance policies, especially long-term care policies, need scrutiny by an informed individual capable of reading such contracts. Funeral ideas may have already been analyzed by friends of your loved one, but these ideas may need to be documented.

In the following pages, each of these subjects will be addressed in detail. Detail is the explicit word now. You can't "kind of know" what the balance in the checkbook is. And the doctor needs to know who has the medical POA should a hospital visit occur. (A flash drive containing this information is a good idea, but be sure it's password protected.) The team should already have been working on the Master Checklist spreadsheet, because now the completed version should be ready to share. My assumption is that this spreadsheet has been customized to fit your particular needs. I'm proud of this beginner's guide. I also know it is only a guide. Mostly, I hope it helps.

Although I have placed this discussion toward the latter part of this book, you might remember that it was Step Two for our team. The external trigger of our father's death moved us into action mode. It paved the way for our long-term plan for our mother, and it made us aware of the need to begin collecting essential paperwork. In many cases, my senior move management business was able to accomplish the move for the senior because the family could present us with the POA. And it was heartwarming to see the level of trust shared by these families.

Fiscal, legal, insurance, and final considerations all need to be assimilated gradually. It's going to take a lot of time to complete this step in your plan. Take the time to collect your essential paperwork, then place it in a fireproof safe. And thank your loved one for reminding you that we should all be doing these same tasks; every family member can benefit from this advice.

The best-case scenario shows that your loved one has carefully placed all these items, including the will and the deeds to any properties, in a safe deposit box. It is a good place to start.

MASTER LIST WITH PROVIDER DECISIONS

ACTIVITY	FAMILY MEMBER	PROVIDER	PHONE/EMAIL
HEALTH COMPANION			
CHOICES FOR REHAB (3)			
VISIT AND/OR INTERVIEW			
VISIT AND/OR INTERVIEW			
CHOICES FOR HOME CARE (3)			
VISIT AND/OR INTERVIEW			
VISIT AND/OR INTERVIEW			
CLEANING PERSON REGULAR			
ESTATE ATTORNEY			
FINANCIAL ADVISOR			
CPA			
SENIOR LIVING COMMUNITIES (3)			
VISIT AND/OR INTERVIEW			
VISIT AND/OR INTERVIEW			
SENIOR MOVE MANAGER			
REALTOR			
GUN SELLER			
JEWELRY BUYER			
COINS/PRECIOUS METALS			
FUNERAL DIRECTOR			
CLEANING PERSON: DEEP APPRAISER			
AUCTION HOUSE			
ESTATE SALES COMPANY			
DONATION PICKUP			
JUNK REMOVAL			

FINANCE COLLECTION

For those of you who decided to jump ahead to this page, I get it. You want to get started, and the finances are where you want to start. The unpaid bills have concerned you, but they have also scared you. You're in I-have-to-fix-this mode. But slow down. The most direct way to help is to get an agreement to have a joint checking account. And the only way to do this is with the explicit consent of your loved one. So go back and read the chapters about the "Senior Conversation" and "Making the Team." I can't emphasize enough that the team approach is the ultimate solution.

Now the extremely necessary discussion about getting the finances in order commences. Initially, I would provide my senior clients with an expandable file system, with prewritten labels such as *Checking/Savings/CD Account(s)*, *Brokerage Account(s)*, *Taxes*, and *Prepaid Receipt(s)*. We'll be analyzing each of these subjects in the following paragraphs. Initially, this task may seem more difficult than it really is. Paperwork needs to be collected and organized. Being detail oriented is the main prerequisite.

Back to the concern about unpaid bills. We're still taking care of the person, but the time has come to begin shared control of the finances. For many family teams, this will become Step One. The team member willing to handle the finances has to offer to help the senior. Usually, your loved one will have very strong opinions about who this should be. Control will be shared for the immediate future.

Checking/Savings/CD Account(s)

Let's begin with the checkbook. Where is it? What bank? You might ask, "Can I help you balance it once a month?" In today's world, paying bills is usually accomplished through the autopay option your bank provides. Check to make sure this is happening. Ask about passwords. And ask about visiting the banker and/or financial advisor to add your emergency contact information. Your concerns about timely payment can and should be a touchy subject. Building confidence with password sharing will come over time. Move forward in the most appropriate manner, and as slowly as necessary.

Balancing the checkbook once a month will provide a good look at how your loved one is handling life. The deposits will reveal income from Social Security, pensions, and annuities. It will also serve as an opening for a review of credit card statements. Doing these reviews together may reveal missing checks and questionable payments. But it can also reveal that an unpaid bill was simply a mistake. And while mistakes happen, we all feel better for the knowing.

As shared control occurs, several other big questions come into focus: How is the account titled? And how should the account be titled in case your loved one becomes incapacitated? (This applies to brokerage accounts as well.) Depending on state law, there are several ownership options. The three common terminologies include: joint account, transfer on death (TOD is how this is shown on the physical check), and a trust.

It's time to consider joint account issues. My husband (a financial advisor since 1980) reminds me that if anything happens to him, my first stop should be the bank. Why? Because in our state, joint bank account assets are frozen upon notice of death. He also advises cleaning out the safe deposit box; another good place to start. Do you have a safe deposit box? Can the finance team member become an authorized signer? Can this person have a key?

TOD accounts are useful because your money is still available to someone else if you die. My consulting company monies were titled this way. If something happened to me, I wanted my husband to be able to get the money. If the checking account is meant to cover operating expenses, payable on death (POD) is a viable option. Just remember that titling an account this way generally means only one team member receives the total amount when the primary owner dies. You can never be too safe when it comes to finances.

Trusts

Trusts, both revocable and irrevocable, should be used when the total of your loved one's assets reach the million-dollar level. Are you laughing? Did you include the value of the house? Real estate values can place you in the millionaire bracket without you realizing it. If you qualify (and even if you don't), consider setting up a trust. My family was surprised to learn that our mother had savings accounts in so many places that the correct solution was to set up a trust. The task of getting all these savings and CDs titled correctly took some time. My mother accomplished this on her own and was quite proud of herself. Except there was one thirty-thousand-dollar CD account that the bank had her set up at age eighty-five, without a beneficiary! So much for avoiding probate, but more about that in the "Legal Collection."

Brokerage account(s)

Not everyone has a brokerage account, but find out if one exists. Your parents' simple life might have you believe that they don't have any money. So where did that thirty-thousand-dollar surprise I just mentioned come from? I'm not sure. What I do know is that parents who lived through the Depression learned all about saving. Several families I worked with were amazed by just how well their parents had saved for a comfortable future.

Taxes and prepaid receipts:

For all taxes, find them and file them. Old income taxes can be fun to look at as income amounts were pretty small by today's standards. While identifying prepaid receipts, be sure to look for preplanned funeral services. Save these items for perusal at a future time.

We've covered a lot of information in this section, so let's review what we've accomplished.

- JOINT ACCESS TO FINANCIAL RECORDS.

- SHARED PASSWORDS FOR ONLINE PAYMENTS.

- EMERGENCY CONTACT INFO ON *ALL* ACCOUNTS.

- ACCESS TO THE SAFE DEPOSIT BOX.

Everyone should be feeling better about the status quo. What a team accomplishment!

FINANCIAL DOCUMENTS

File:

- BANK CHECKING ACCOUNTS: JOINT, POD, TRUST

- BANK SAVINGS ACCOUNTS: JOINT, POD, TRUST

- BANK CDS: MUST HAVE BENEFICIARY; JOINT, POD, TRUST

- BROKERAGE ACCOUNTS: JOINT, POD, TRUST, IRA

- PASSWORD JOURNAL

- RECEIPTS FOR PREPLANNED FUNERAL SERVICES

- TAXES: PAST SEVEN YEARS

- TRUSTS

Income items

- ANNUITY PAYMENTS

- SOCIAL SECURITY PAYMENTS

- PENSION PAYMENTS

Expense items

- CREDIT CARD STATEMENTS

- MORTGAGE PAYMENTS

- CAR PAYMENTS

Other

- SOCIAL SECURITY DEATH BENEFIT

- OTHER DEBTS

LEGAL COLLECTION

As we finish our discussion on the finance collection, we immediately begin our discussion on the legal collection. There is some overlap here. The overlap between legal and financial concerns consists of *trusts, powers of attorney* (POAs), and *advance directives*. Items that fall into a mainly legal category are *wills, deeds,* and *titles.* In my mind, these divisions fall into help for the living, then help for the survivors. In case you haven't noticed, I'm always concerned with helping the living senior first. To that end, this discussion begins with POAs and ends with the will.

As you might conclude, one team member needs to find a good estate attorney in the state where your loved one resides (estate laws vary by state, an extremely important consideration). Ask your CPA and your financial advisor for recommendations. They become involved in these situations out of necessity. The referral network among these professions is a constant. Having lived with a financial advisor for forty-plus years, I have overheard many conversations revolving around estate planning. Use this resource wisely. It has the benefit of allowing you to interact with the professionals chosen by your loved one. Evaluate them as you ask for their help; it's a better starting place than going it alone.

Power of Attorney (POA)

POA is short for *power of attorney*. It is a term you hear quite often in your caregiving role. What it means is that your loved one is relying on you to make decisions for them. Their best interest is assumed to be fully understood by you. However, in my experience, a POA also assumes that you can communicate with your loved one better than others can. At times, decisions can be discussed then mutually agreed upon. I can still see a dutiful daughter seeking her father's agreement about what to do with her mother's (his spouse's) art pieces. The POA gave her the right to dispose of those pieces as she saw fit, and her heart gave her the compassion to share that decision-making. This type of interaction should be emulated whenever possible—POA, tempered with concern for the living.

Sharing POAs is possible, but not recommended. However, there are two kinds of POAs. The POA described above is mainly for financial items. It lets you take over all financial aspects of your loved one's life, from paying bills to using funds available for any purposes you might deem necessary. Remodeling the house with ramps and safety bars and paying for moving expenses are good examples of life-enhancing choices. I'm sure you will discover other good examples as you fulfill your POA duties.

The other POA that can be shared is the medical POA (sometimes referred to as the *power to pull the plug*.) Ideally, this POA should be given to the team member with a medical background or access to medical advice. What it means is that your loved one is relying on you to make medical decisions. My family has two nurses, so they shared the medical POA. Questioning why your loved one is having surgery, at any age, is appropriate. Having someone you can call who can explain it to you is better. Be aware of the burden you carry when you accept this role. Life and death decisions may be in your future.

Advance Directive

There are several forms of advance directives. "A written statement of a person's wishes regarding medical treatment" is the dictionary definition. A medical POA is one form; living wills and DNRs are variations on the same idea. The concept is to allow people to designate their wishes should they become incapacitated. The biggest advantage of advance directives is that they provide the questions you should be asking. Our state has an advance directive, printed on yellow paper, which was designed by estate attorneys. The questions included document your wishes on feeding tubes and breathing machines (not the same as oxygen concentrators). Thoughtful, sensitive decision-making is its goal, and it seems to be working. In some instances, the DNR has been replaced by this more comprehensive form. Thank you to estate attorneys for their proactive stance.

Do Not Resuscitate Order (DNR)

What do you know about DNRs? A do not resuscitate order is often taped on the inside door of the room in senior living residences. It explicitly tells everyone your wishes, especially if you are incapacitated. (There are now medical alert bracelets and necklaces that provide the same information.) It lets emergency workers know that the use of artificial life support, such as cardiopulmonary resuscitation (CPR), is declined because this individual prefers a natural death.

A personal example is my nephew, aged twenty-one, who had to share his mother's wishes with the medical staff. My husband, after his mother's fall and the resulting brain hemorrhage, shared his mother's wishes. Being in "control" of death decisions is hard on that person. Be ready to offer emotional support. Knowing that you have talked about the arrival of a day like this is comforting. You need to know you did the right thing.

Reality check: You walk in and find your loved one on the floor. What are you going to do? You're going to call 911. You're going to say that there is a DNR. They will come to evaluate the health of your loved one. You are strong in saying no CPR. The emergency workers are the professionals. They will advise you. They will offer choices. More than likely, you will choose the hospital. Give yourself time to make an informed decision. Then try to be realistic about the results. You accepted the medical role, but now you're not sure what to do. Calling your team members will be necessary, anyway, so why not share the burden? Keep reminding yourself that dying is the final step in life. Celebrate knowing and sharing this person's story. It's as OK as it can be.

AFTER DEATH

Once your loved one has passed away, the next phase, that is, disposition of assets, can occur. Your estate attorney comes back into the picture now. You'll probably want to be refreshed on what the trust and will say. Be aware that upon death, the POA ends and the will takes over as the legal document. The executor of the will becomes the person in control and the person designated to make financial decisions. If the POA and the executor are the same, there is little controversy. This issue was probably already addressed by your estate attorney.

What can happen if the POA and the executor are different people?

A client died while we were selling some of her memorabilia. We had been given permission by the POA to sell everything. The executor insisted that she didn't want anything sold until she could see it first. Luckily, a check for the proceeds of sales had already been cut. Since the sales preceded death, the POA was the legal document involved. Although the executor had the right to stop current and future sales, completed sales could not be reversed. Another lesson learned.

Dying Without a Will

What can happen if you die without a will (legally called intestate)? If your team doesn't take care of this in advance, control passes to the state where the deceased last had a legal residence. Probate is your individual state's solution to deciding who gets what. And, of course, it comes at a cost. Skip this step and about half of your (yes, your, at this point) assets go to the state and to attorney fees. Attorney fees spent to avoid probate will be less than those spent to title finances correctly, so do it as soon as possible.

Other Assets

Deeds are our next major legal concern. Where is that safe deposit box key again? In many instances, a senior's house is their largest investment. Selling the family home comes with its own set of emotions. Selling it to a family member can be a comfort. Much like in a divorce, the family member buying the house will have to buy out the other members. When possible, give family members time to think through this dilemma.

Given enough time (set a deadline), our nephew realized he couldn't keep a house in a different state. As it turned out, the house was priced correctly (another team member responsibility) and sold quickly.

Titles are our final legal concern—for cars mainly. In order to sell a vehicle, the POA or executor will need the title to the vehicle. It's probably in the safe deposit box, with the will. If you can't find the title, don't be too upset. I've seen this happen many times. The Department of Motor Vehicles in your state has a link just for this situation. Nice to know that it's fairly easy to get a duplicate/replacement title.

A brief review of your legal accomplishments is in order:

- AN ATTORNEY IS FOUND AND "ENGAGED."

- WILLS, TRUSTS, AND POAS ARE PREPARED, SIGNED, AND NOTARIZED.

- AN EXECUTOR IS CHOSEN FOR THE PURPOSE OF HANDLING ASSETS UPON THE DEATH OF YOUR LOVED ONE.

- A POA IS CHOSEN FOR HANDLING ASSETS WHILE YOUR LOVED ONE IS LIVING.

- A MEDICAL POA IS CHOSEN FOR HANDLING HEALTH DECISIONS IF YOUR LOVED ONE IS INCAPACITATED.

It has taken months, but the legal aspects of passing on are now addressed. Please celebrate these accomplishments. There will be more to come. And it is money well spent.

LEGAL DOCUMENTS

Team Member Paperwork Needed to Help the Living

- POWER OF ATTORNEY (POA) FOR FINANCIAL DECISIONS

- ADVANCE DIRECTIVE

- MEDICAL POWER OF ATTORNEY (MD POA) FOR HEALTH DECISIONS

- LIVING WILL

- DO NOT RESUSCITATE (DNR)

- TRUST

- YOUR OWN LIST OF WHO GETS WHAT

Team Member Paperwork Needed after Death

- WILL

- DEED(S)

- TITLE(S) TO CARS

- COPIES OF DEATH CERTIFICATE (AT LEAST TEN)

- YOUR OWN LIST OF WHO GETS WHAT

INSURANCE

Insurance is, by definition, "a company guarantee of compensation in return for payment of a premium."

Insurance has become a necessary part of our existence. Health insurance for those sixty-five and older is handled by Medicare and Medicare Advantage plans. Although there are a few other alternatives, Medicare is basically required as soon as one reaches the magic number of sixty-five. Long-term care insurance can be a great resource if you already have it, but the cost is almost prohibitive. Life insurance can also be a great resource for additional monies. Asking your loved one questions about insurance policies can be fairly easy. This type of easy discussion might be a great lead-in for more difficult discussions about financial and legal matters.

Medicare for All sounds like a great idea. Let me share my experience with it. First of all, Medicare is *not* free; it is taken out of your Social Security monies. Was I surprised? You bet. Medicare pays for just about every test your doctor orders. That's the good news. But is it really? The team member with the medical POA will be taking control of your medical tests. This team decision maker will determine whether tests ordered by the doctor should be taken.

For example, my uncle had a test for his heart, which required a dye to be used. This dye caused his kidneys to fail. That's right. While his heart remained the same, the new status for his kidneys meant he was on dialysis for the rest of his life. Did Medicare pay for all of this? Yes. Did Medicare improve his quality of life? No. The importance of the medical team member is indeed critical. Cost is only one issue for a well-lived life.

Medicare Advantage plans are designed to take care of what original Medicare doesn't. My experience with this extra level of insurance is limited. I can remember examining every one of my mom's Blue Cross Blue Shield statements. And you know, they were all accurate. No outstanding bills to worry about even though she spent around four years in memory care.

Long-term care insurance, as I saw my clients struggling with it, is extremely hard to decipher. For one thing, long-term care premiums are not fixed; in other words, they can (and do) change almost annually. Review such policies with both financial and legal team members present. A trusted insurance agent (not the one who is selling you such a policy) can explain the details in this meeting. In addition to cost, my clients' children often complained about the waiting period before a long-term care policy "kicked in." Is a ninety-day waiting period realistic? Many times the client passed away during that waiting period. Was the cost/benefit worth it? I can't answer that question, but financial and legal team members can help you with this important discussion and decision.

Life, homeowner, renter, and auto insurance policies all need to be carefully held in your files. Life insurance requires a beneficiary. Ideally, when the trust was being set up your estate attorney had you complete the paperwork to make the trust the life insurance beneficiary. Homeowner, renter, and auto insurance will need to be canceled as these items become unnecessary. Usernames and passwords are needed to make these changes. After death, copies of the death certificate may be required for cancellation, but not always.

INSURANCE POLICIES

- HEALTH

- MEDICARE

- MEDICARE ADVANTAGE

- LONG-TERM CARE

- DISABILITY

- LIFE

- HOMEOWNER

- RENTER

- AUTO

PREPAID FUNERAL SERVICES

Finding the joy in a life well lived is the true intent behind memorial services, thus the commonly used designation of a "celebration of life." Many details are considered when planning this celebration. Try to think of this final event the same way you think of weddings or graduations. You want the day to be perfect. You can't do it over. So much emotion is going to be shared again and again. Looking it at it this way, it makes perfect sense to do as much planning as possible to get it right.

In getting it right, it helps to understand that, in addition to commemorating the life of the deceased, the living need a place and a time to grieve. We all need time to accept the inevitable—time to process the finality of death. While we can still "talk" to the deceased, it's not really the same. We say, "Wish you were here."

For my family team, the prepaid funeral decision became the pre-planned funeral decision. Our father's funeral had walked us through the steps while we were grieving. It didn't give us time to plan perfectly. And, since he had terminal cancer, we had time to plan.

Will this be your Step One? Have you had the "Senior Conversation"?

After our father's death, our mother decided she needed to be ready for her own death. Even though she passed away some twenty years later, it was a comfort to have gone through those decisions with her ahead of time.

The funeral director, at the request of our mother, took the lead role. His business-like questions were welcomed for this visit. The funeral home would be the same one we had used for our father. Choice of casket was easier, as we had already gone through that process. Choice of prayer cards meant looking at their selection (twenty years later, the same selection wasn't available). Burial would be at the same cemetery, in the family plot, next to our father. The church service would also be at the same location. Contact numbers were exchanged. Step One for our team was complete.

When someone you know dies is the perfect time to start talking about funerals in general. This external trigger can be the impetus for things the family can preplan: burial clothes, music, and videos. In my personal as well as my business life, burial clothes have been important. Who doesn't want to look their best for their final exit? Taking note of favorite songs is always joyful. Prepare a list for the church service as well as the reception. When we heard the Eagles at a recent reception, we had to smile at how appropriate this type of music was for this motorcycle adventurer. My organ-playing, traditional Baptist friend would much prefer "How Great Thou Art." Video ideas will be many, so they are presented in "Recording the Legacy."

As you attend services for friends and relatives, begin making mental notes of what you would want or *not* want when the time comes. There will be additional things to consider, such as choosing a minister and other potential speakers. Choices and decisions on possible dates and times, as well as locations, will be made by your family team, then published. Memorial service handouts will be printed listing your preplanned, agreed-upon music. Food for the reception and number of possible attendees all need to be considered. Did we ever decide if the estate was paying for relatives to attend?

We are all given a finite time to live on this earth. Preparing the structure for the inevitable end-of-life celebration is right in front of you. Seize the moment. Prepare concrete plans. Making the funeral a prepaid event makes sense. Make sure the team member responsible for finances has a copy of the receipt. Small decisions like these open the door to the end-of-life decision-making. It all begins with a first step. And the acknowledgment that we are in this together.

A concise list of details follows.

FUNERAL BASICS

Prearranged Decisions

- FUNERAL HOME PROVIDER:

  - CASKET OR URN

  - OPEN/CLOSED CASKET OR CREMATION

- PLACE OF MEMORIAL SERVICE

- BURIAL SITE

- PRAYER CARDS (SENIORS KEEP A LOT OF THESE)

- GUEST BOOK REGISTER

Individual wishes

- ORGAN/TISSUE DONATION

- BURIAL CLOTHES

- SONGS

- AUDIO/VIDEO OF PHOTOS

- PAYING FOR RELATIVES TO ATTEND

At death

- CONTACT FUNERAL HOME

- CONTACT MINISTER/CHURCH

- DECIDE ON TYPE OF SERVICE

- DECIDE/PUBLISH DATE, TIME, PLACE OF MEMORIAL SERVICE

- PREPARE LIST OF SPEAKERS/READERS

- PREPARE MEMORIAL SERVICE HANDOUTS

- PREPARE SONGS FOR SERVICE/RECEPTION

- UPDATE AUDIO/VIDEO OF PHOTOS

- PUBLISH OBITUARY (WITH SUGGESTIONS ON FLOWERS AND/OR DONATIONS)

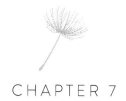

CHAPTER 7

~~~~~~~~~

RECORDING
THE LEGACY

"The Story of My Loved One" is a better way to describe what will be accomplished in this section. Seniors, as elderly members of the team, can begin their unique prewritten obituary. Storytelling members of the team can use their skills to begin composing the personal history, aka "His Story/Her Story." Those family team members with an artistic bent should be recruited to begin the photo and ephemera collection. Photos, drawings, and anything handwritten are an incredible source for personal history. How do you think your loved one wants to be remembered? How does your loved one want to be remembered? These are two very different questions, with possibly different answers.

What unique experiences can be recaptured to describe the unique person to be commemorated? Does asking how the holidays were celebrated when your loved ones were little often bring a smile? Capture that moment. National historical questions are always intriguing. What do you remember about 9/11? This question, to an American, brings an almost immediate response. We all remember exactly where we were and exactly what we were doing. The Challenger explosion and the Kennedy assassination are two more examples of national events that created personal emotional responses.

Local history is important as well. What buildings became part of the National Register of Historic Places? Do you remember how that happened? And family stories have an equally important role for events to be shared by survivors. You were bitten by a dog! That explains a lot.

During the course of my eleven years serving the senior community, I met so many wonderful people and heard so many wonderful stories. There are two client stories involving national historical events that I feel compelled to share as unique examples.

The Pearl Harbor survivor is my first one. After helping this man and his family several times, he confided that he survived the December 7, 1941 attack by taking his sixteen-year-old self into the dugout on the baseball field. He admitted that the dugout was already pretty crowded by the time he got there. His quick thinking saved his life. The regret I heard in his telling reminded me of the regret I had heard in my father's telling of not being chosen to serve in the military during WWII. This man's daughter, and I, would likely not be here had circumstances been different.

Another compelling example concerns the 1918 flu pandemic, aka the Spanish flu. While I was helping my client move, she shared a story about how she was raised by her grandmother. She said she didn't really remember her mother; she was told her mother died walking home from work. She said a lot of people died that way right after the Great War (WWI). Curiosity led me to the discovery of the 1918 pandemic—a piece of history I hadn't even known existed. My client's reaction to reading the printed account of this piece of history still makes me emotional. She started crying. "I always thought my mother didn't want me," she said.

We can learn so much from these individual histories. Most important, the stories are a good way to start having the "Senior Conversation." Make these stories the beginning point for remembering; as more stories emerge, weave them into the family memories. Life's journey takes all of us in different directions, defining us as individuals. There is so much to learn from our seniors before they pass away. Take the time now to listen, to learn, then to pass along these poignant moments in your own history.

In preparing a class on writing an obituary, I prepared the exercise "If I Die Today." Its design encourages a long-term overview of life. Write the first thing that comes into your mind; it will help you describe what makes the person you see in the mirror each morning so special. And the obituary, memorial service, and eulogy will reflect it as well.

If I Die Today

If I die today,
Remember me as the young girl with buck teeth,
Body surfing at the beach,
Running into a stingray.

Remember me as the high school ...

EXAMPLE 1:..

EXAMPLE 2:..

EXAMPLE 3:..

If I die today,
Remember me at my best as a mother of two,
Nurturing, teaching, loving each and every moment,
Turning daughters into strong women.

Remember me as ...

EXAMPLE 1:..

EXAMPLE 2:..

EXAMPLE 3:..

If I die today,

Remember me as a friend to few,

Because true friendship requires listening with your heart,

And sharing your heart's love is not limitless.

Remember me as an active ...

EXAMPLE 1:..

EXAMPLE 2:..

EXAMPLE 3:..

If I die today,

Remember me as an agent of change,

Building a business to help seniors and their families,

Understanding the challenges of moving a lifetime.

Remember me as an author,

Giving light to dying thoughts,

Opening the door to discussions on dying well.

And when I die,

Remember the good times, and let the others go.

PREWRITTEN OBITUARY

Did you know that famous people always have prewritten obituaries? I stumbled upon this fact one day as I was looking for Paul Bocuse, who wasn't dead at the time. As a writer, it makes perfect sense to me to prepare a synopsis ahead of time. By writing an obituary before it's needed, two things are accomplished: an interesting obituary, and relieving other family members of a duty difficult to perform upon a loved one's death.

First, realize that there are two types of obituaries: the official one for the news and the personal one for the memorial service.

The official one is meant to be brief and factual; it lists everything one needs to know in a standard format. A fee is charged to publish in traditional and online newspapers, so keep it to one hundred words. Complete the "Prewritten Obituary Basics" on the following page. Place it in a separate file on your computer (Before the Time Comes). Print it, then file it with the essential paperwork. Retrieve this information and update it as needed. Since smartphones are essentially address books as well, place the phone's password in this same location.

A published obituary with the place and time of the funeral brings comfort to those who wish to make a final visit. It allows time to adjust schedules or send flowers or donations. Personal calls or texts after a loved one's death are difficult. Being able to direct friends and relatives to a common listing relieves some of the family's stress. The official obituary ensures that facts are easily accessible. Reading about it, in print, makes it more concrete. It finalizes the death announcement.

What Do I Want My Family to Remember Me For?

The personal obituary is where your unique character can shine through. Make it interesting.

We've briefly touched on this topic in our past discussions. This is an opportunity to tell the story of you. Were you funny? Did people want to listen to your stories? Did you travel a lot? Why not list some of your most memorable trips and conclude by saying, "I finally came to rest here. And I won't be going anywhere else." Birth and death dates, as well as the names of surviving members of the family, should still be included.

Since this is a team effort, the opportunity for other family members to gather their thoughts can occur at this same time. Who is considering composing a eulogy? Remembering good times has been part of discussions for "Recording the Legacy." What stories might be shared? If emotions allow, will the joy shine through? Not too somber, not too serious—a true celebration of life.

"Mom, Wife, Business Owner … Hiker, Runner, Traveler, Reader, Lover of Life."

These are some sentiments my husband included in a picture bio for me on my sixtieth birthday.

"Grandmama, Author." These are some other successes I would add to that list.

Music

Music is one thing that surrounds our lives yet seems to be in the background. Music, at the memorial service, comes into the foreground and tugs at our heartstrings. Choose these songs ahead of time; choose the organist and the soloist during this same time. Place these selections in the computer file and the printed file. These choices, combined with the other choices made here, describe a unique person. As Cat Stevens wrote, "If You Want to Sing Out, Sing Out.".

PREWRITTEN OBITUARY BASICS

Full Name:...

(PHOTO)

Date of Birth (Month/Day/YYYY):...

Survived by:...

....

In Lieu of Flowers (charity/donation): ....

....

Place of Memorial (name/addess):...

....

Place of Reception (name/addess):...

....

Interesting Characteristics:

Loved to do: ....

Remembered for: ....

....

HIS STORY/HER STORY

Regrets and successes define each of us. Using the "Senior Con-versation" as a starting point, the listener on the team can initiate a discussion about regrets as well as successes. This order is important because so much can be learned from mistakes and failures. The knowledge gained from such hard lessons often leads to maturity and success. Listening is an art. Storytelling is an art. Personal stories will be retold again and again at family gatherings when recorded appropriately. Take the time to develop these skills of listening and storytelling. The reward for your family will be immeasurable.

Regrets

Regrets are do-overs. If you had the chance to do something dif-ferently, what would it be? If you believe that everything happens for a reason, you shouldn't have many regrets. So listen carefully now. Hold on to your "but" until the regret is fully described. This is probably a story that hasn't been told too many times. A miscar-riage, a family member with mental illness, and dealing with alcohol-ism are some examples that come to mind. Life is far from perfect. Regrets have a place in each personal story. Measure their impor-tance. Adversities help to define the person your loved one became. Treasure this confidence.

In the introduction to this section, the concept of regrets and their consequences was presented using two client examples. On a per-sonal level, the discovery of my mother's letter to the Veterans Admin-istration led our family to understand why she was so strongly inde-pendent. She regretted that her brothers were sent to an orphanage while she was able to live with her aunt and uncle. The consequence for her children was the lesson to plan ahead and to rely fiercely on yourself. Regrets and consequences distilled into making us all who we are today.

Successes

Successes are much easier to treasure. Many of the women I had the pleasure to move were "telephone ladies" and switchboard operators. Working outside the home was less common in the 1900s. This shared experience has led these women to gather for monthly luncheons. They see themselves as so much more than "red hat" ladies. This pride is an outward representation of their success.

If you're interested in history, personal accounts of historical events can be remarkable. Most of us can remember 9/11. What strong emotions we all shared as Americans on that day. Our seniors have many more examples to share of such moments. The seniors I moved were shaped by World War II, the Great Depression, and even World War I (aka the Great War). In moving "my seniors," I also met and moved two seniors who had combined their efforts and saved an important local school building.

Use the "Remember When" questions on the next page to start the flow of memories. Ask, listen, record. Bringing historical events alive like this transforms them into reality and secures them in our minds. A sense of being there and understanding what it was like to live in that different time is one more treasure for families.

Personal stories about family members are also fun. These easy talks get the memory juices flowing. Learning to ride a bike, eating at Grandma's house, and Sunday drives are all simple subjects, important only to your family. Take stock of these stories as they become part of the fabric of the family.

These discussions are often enjoyable. My brother recently shared such a story about fishing with my father. To hear his version of fishing (which was, to me, a boring waste of time) was such a surprise; I'll always remember his laughter in the telling. Joy is what I feel when I hear his voice in my head.

Remember the good times and let the others go. This is a sentiment I write on cards sent to those going through a death in the family. Celebrate your loved one's legacy.

"REMEMBER WHEN" QUESTIONS

Family

- HOW DID YOU AND GRANDDADDY (GRANDMA) MEET?

- DO YOU REMEMBER YOUR FIRST-GRADE TEACHER?

- HOW OLD WERE YOU WHEN YOU LEFT HOME?

- TELL ME ABOUT THE DAY I WAS BORN.

- WHERE HAVE YOU TRAVELED AND WHY?

Local Historical Events

- MY TEACHER SAYS THE CITY BURNED DOWN IN 1904. WHAT HAPPENED?

- HOW DID YOU SAVE YOUR ELEMENTARY SCHOOL FROM BEING TORN DOWN?

- WHY DO WE HAVE A ST. PATRICK'S DAY PARADE?

- WHY DO WE HAVE A RODEO PARADE?

National Historical Events (Use a search engine and your own date range)

- WHAT IS A "VICTORY GARDEN"?

- CAN YOU TELL ME ABOUT THE VIETNAM WAR?

- WHERE WERE YOU WHEN PRESIDENT KENNEDY WAS KILLED?

- WHAT CAN YOU TELL ME ABOUT THE SPACE PROGRAM?

- DO YOU REMEMBER THE BERLIN WALL? WHAT WAS THAT ABOUT?

PHOTO AND EPHEMERA COLLECTION

What should follow the discovery of something that made your loved one the person they eventually became? Who can take the photos acquired over a lifetime and turn them into the family history? What happens to handwritten letters and recipes? Is anyone interested in genealogy? What exactly are these awards? Newspaper clippings? An address book? Prayer cards? What should follow the discovery of something that made your loved one the person they eventually became? This is another good place to start "Recording the Legacy."

When the time came to clear out my mother's house, the task of reviewing the paperwork became mine. Why? Because I lived far away, and this seemed like the best way for me to help. Two checked bags and a carry-on contained my family assignment. I had no idea how to proceed. As it turned out, it took me several years to complete this assignment. (Actually, I arrived at a certain point, then passed one suitcase on to my nephew. I had done as much as I cared to do.) Mentioning this dilemma is my way of giving you permission to be imperfect.

Creating order out of the chaos of saved photos creates the possibility of seeing a person more clearly. In today's world, with point-and-shoot camera phones and cloud storage, the number of photos has skyrocketed, making it even harder to arrive at someone's true nature. (Check the number of pictures on your phone and then write down the time period that covers. Crazy, right?) My clients' grandchildren were the family members most likely to organize these memories. Photo-book software and photo-quality scanners are the tools available to create memory books. Videos and slide shows make memories come alive. Start with a goal of a maximum of five photos per year. (Age times five equals?) The family can enjoy them now, then use them for the memorial service later.

Include Ephemera

But true memory books need to incorporate the addition of ephemera, that is, all the other "finds" included in your paperwork organization. Handwritten letters deserve special consideration in any family history. A recent relocation uncovered the existence of the correspondence between a son and his father after WWI. Written on onionskin airmail paper, it told of how the son had spent those final historic days. My husband's grandfather wrote those words in 1919. In 2019, his grandson (my husband) visited the locations in France named in that letter—one hundred years later.

Awards and medals have also earned their place in the family history. Living in a military town means a lot of military medals and insignias came my way. Awards for athletic achievements (mutton busting?), for marathons, and for senior games were among this same collection. And a surprising number of awards for work on the space program made my work with these seniors more significant.

Handwritten recipes, actually any family recipes, make ephemera collection a joy. Three-by-five-inch notecard boxes still grace the kitchens of many seniors. Recipes for Christmas cookies are especially enjoyable. "Connoisseur Casserole" and "Philippine Spareribs" will be among my family's recipe treasures. Family cookbooks are another type of memory book, easily achievable with modern electronic tools.

One more thought on these personal collections: dispose of them in a respectful manner. When clients asked me to put photo books and genealogy records in the dumpster, I couldn't do it. How to handle military medals was also something I found an alternative solution for. Your respect has guided you to complete this family history project. Letting go of the collection is the final phase.

PHOTO CATEGORIES

- FAMILY

- TRAVEL

- HOBBIES

- OTHER

EPHEMERA CATEGORIES

- ART/DRAWINGS

- AWARDS AND MEDALS

- GENEALOGY RECORDS

- CARDS:

    - HOLIDAY CARDS

    - SPECIAL DAY CARDS

    - PRAYER CARDS

- HANDWRITTEN ITEMS

- LETTERS

- RECIPES

CHAPTER 8

CONCLUSION

've spent a lot of time crying while writing this book. My assumption is that you have done the same, at times, while reading it.

I remember giving my mother baths, dressed in my bathing suit, in a handicap-accessible hotel room in Ocean City, Maryland. I remember taking her to eat oysters at Phillips on the Beach, and surreptitiously telling the server to continue bringing more until she stopped eating. For some reason, these memories haven't gotten easier over time.

What has gotten easier is that I know I did my best. If you have spent the time to read this entire book, rest assured that you, too, have done your best.

Take the advice presented in this book and use it. Complete any and all of the worksheets. Each small step accomplished brings the family one step closer to an easier transition to the final chapter of life. Embrace the simplicity of the five essentials presented in this book:

- MAKING A PLAN

- CHOOSING A NEW HOME

- TAKING CARE OF THE PERSON

- COLLECTING ESSENTIAL PAPERWORK

- RECORDING THE LEGACY

As much as possible, I hope you have seen a way to transform the maze of Before the Time Comes responsibilities into a straight path. Pass this wisdom on to those who need it.

A VIEW OF THE ESSENTIALS

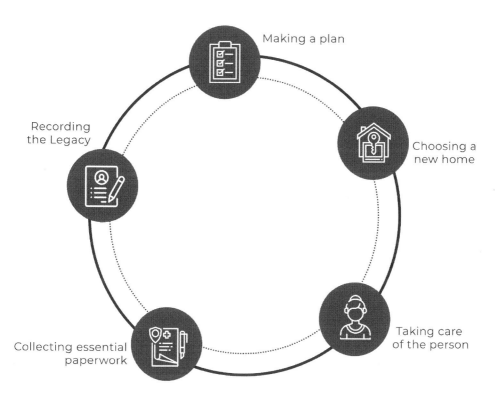

Making a plan

Choosing a
new home

Taking care
of the person

Collecting essential
paperwork

Recording
the Legacy

ACKNOWLEDGMENTS

Without the 1,000-plus families who committed themselves to my company's care, I would not have a foundation for writing this book. To all of you, I am extremely grateful. The lessons learned are contained in this book. Thank you.

Community partners were also very helpful. They recognized the value of an outsider like my company taking family concerns and putting them first. A gradual melding of business and family concerns is what made these partnerships a success. A special shout-out to Marsha for her unwavering commitment to what was a novel concept in 2005. She told all her potential residents that I would replace the "Where do I start?" question with an action plan. This book takes that same approach. Thank you also to Jo, Mark, Shirley, Donna, Jeanine, Echo, and Connie as well as Angela, Lorelei, and John—sales personnel at the various communities. Your understanding of how to help seniors is reflected in these pages.

Employees are the heart of any business. So thank you to my best workers, Margo, Betty, and Jamie.

NASMM's annual conferences provided opportunities to share ideas as well as improve business practices. Thank you, Mary Kay and Jennifer.

To my friends: Donna—thank you for being my thought leader; Linda, fellow author—thank you for all your insights on publishing; Devon, fellow author—thank you for all your counseling.

To my beta readers: Michele, my niece, and Michael, my nephew—your changes are included. Many thanks.

To my reviewer(s): Jackie—so glad you saw the value of this book immediately.

To my family: Jim, Wendy, Cheryl, and the sisters—Ellen, Agnes, Mary, Cathy, Marian—for the countless number of times you read, reread, and listened—thank you.

To the readers of this book: any author needs *you*, the *reader*, so thank you for reading.

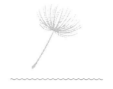

ABOUT
MONICA YOUNG

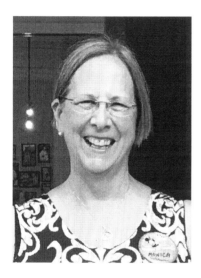

I n 2005, the need to help senior citizens negotiate the later stages of life led Monica Young to create her own senior move manager business (SMM). Her involvement in this industry has included presenting at national conferences, participating as a panelist for "Ask the Expert," and serving as a board member for the National Association of Senior Move Managers (NASMM) from 2013 to 2015.

On the national level, Monica's business earned the A+ certification (one of the top twenty-five in the nation); on the local level, her business was recognized in 2016 as a Joe Henjum Senior Accolades nominee. After eleven years and 1000-plus moves, she sold the business to a national organization.

Now, to further share her capacity to help seniors and their families, Monica has embarked on her newest career as author.

Her life's journey has included working in the transportation department at Walt Disney World in Florida during its opening months and fund-raising for the United States Air Force Academy's Association of Graduates in Colorado Springs. She currently lives with her husband in the foothills of the Sangre de Cristo Mountains and travels as often as possible.

•

Made in the USA
Columbia, SC
17 August 2020